HOSPITAL and CLINICAL PHARMACY

PRACTICAL NOTEBOOK

for

Final Year Diploma in Pharmacy

(According to the new syllabus prescribed by the Pharmacy Council of India, Education Regulation 1991, implemented in the year 1993, for Diploma in Pharmacy Students)

Varun Dutt Sharma M. Pharm.
Principal

S.K. Pandey B. Pharm.
Sr. Lecturer

Janta Polytechnic, Jahangirabad, Bulandshahar, Uttar Pradesh

CBS

CBS Publishers & Distributors Pvt. Ltd.

New Delhi • Bengaluru • Chennai • Kochi • Kolkata • Mumbai
Hyderabad • Nagpur • Patna • Pune • Vijayawada

Hospital and Clinical Pharmacy
PRACTICAL NOTEBOOK

ISBN: 978-81-239-1424-4

First Edition: 2007
Reprint: 2008, 2011, 2014, 2015, 2017, 2018, 2019, 2020

Published by **Satish Kumar Jain** and produced by **Varun Jain** for
CBS Publishers & Distributors Pvt. Ltd.,
4819/XI Prahlad Street, 24 Ansari Road, Daryaganj, New Delhi - 110002
delhi@cbspd.com, cbspubs@airtelmail.in • www.cbspd.com
Ph.: 23289259, 23266861, 23266867 • Fax: 011-23243014

Corporate Office: 204 FIE, Industrial Area, Patparganj, Delhi - 110 092
Ph: 49344934 • Fax: 011-49344935
E-mail: publishing@cbspd.com • publicity@cbspd.com

Branches:
- ***Bengaluru:*** 2975, 17th Cross, K.R. Road, Bansankari 2nd Stage, Bengaluru - 70 • Ph: +91-80-26771678/79 • Fax: +91-80-26771680 E-mail: cbsbng@gmail.com, bangalore@cbspd.com
- ***Chennai:*** No. 7, Subbaraya Street, Shenoy Nagar, Chennai - 600030 Ph: +91-44-26681266, 26680620 • Fax: +91-44-42032115 E-mail: chennai@cbspd.com
- ***Kochi:*** Ashana House, 39/1904, A.M. Thomas Road, Valanjambalam, Ernakulum, Kochi • Ph: +91-484-4059061-65 Fax: +91-484-4059065 • E-mail: cochin@cbspd.com
- ***Kolkata:*** 6-B, Ground Floor, Rameshwar Shaw Road, Kolkata - 700014 Ph: +91-33-22891126/7/8 • E-mail: kolkata@cbspd.com
- ***Mumbai:*** 83-C, Dr. E. Moses Road, Worli, Mumbai - 400018 Ph: +91-9833017933, 022-24902340/41 • E-mail: mumbai@cbspd.com

Representatives:
- Hyderabad: 0-9885175004
- Patna: 0-9334159340
- Jharkhand: 0-9811541605
- Nagpur: 0-9021734563
- Pune: 0-9623451994
- Uttarakhand: 0-9716462459

Printed at:
India Binding House, Noida, UP (India)

Certificate

Student's Name ____

Class ________________________ Roll No. __________________

This is to certify that experiments, written in the index, have been performed by the student, are satisfactory.

Grade.................. Name and signature of lab. in-charge

College stamp Date ....

Preface

The ultimate objective of technical education is to develop relevant skill, creativity and competency among the students so as to enable them to perform the task effectively and efficiently later in the world of work. Practical work consists of tasks which required some manipulation of apparatus or some action.

To obtain the above aim, and reduces the writing work load to some extent to the students the present practical notebook came in existence. This practical notebook contains 25 exercises from the topics, i.e. preparation of transfusion fluids, testing of raw materials, evaluation of surgical dressings, sterilization of surgical instruments, glassware and other hospital supplies, handling and use of data processing equipments which covers whole syllabus of this subject.

In rapid technological advancement the basic knowledge about the handling of computer is essential because it is used in hospital to maintain records, medical research, drug information, inventory control and patient profile, etc.

Left-hand side page of every exercise has been left blank for calculation, labeling and other information. Few blank pages are provided at the end of this manual, so that students can use these pages for writing additional experiments guided by teachers depending on availability of reagents and infrastructure of concern laboratory.

We shall be gratefully acknowledged the comments, suggestions and criticism by respected teachers and students from the improvement of future edition. We express sincere thanks to Mr Satish Kumar Jain and Mr Y.N. Arjuna, M/S CBS Publishers & Distributors, for their cooperation, encouragement and assistance in bringing out the present form of this practical manual. Finally our greatest gratitude is to our colleagues, friends and family members, etc.

Varun Dutt Sharma • S.K. Pandey

Syllabus

Marks: 100
No of hours: 50

1. Preparation of transfusion fluids.
2. Testing of raw materials used in –1.
3. Evaluation of surgical dressings.
4. Sterilization of surgical instruments, glassware and other hospital supplies.
5. Handling and use of data processing equipments.

Contents

INDEX

S. No.	Name of the experiment	Page No.	Remarks

INDEX

S. No.	Name of the experiment	Page No.	Remarks

1

Preparation of Transfusion Fluids

1. Washing and cleaning of containers and closures

Wash the glass bottles, and rubber closures with detergent, free flowing water followed by rinsing them with water for injection.

2. Drying and sterilization

Sterilize the dried bottles and closures by autoclaving at 121° C for 15 minutes.

3. Weighing of ingredients and mixing

weight the required quantity of ingredient/ingredients and dissolve it /them in sufficient quantity of water for injection to make the solution up to stated volume.

4. Filtration

Filter the above prepared solution with suitable filter media, i.e. sintered glass funnel or bacteria proof membrane filter or Millipore filters, etc.

5. Filling and sealing

Fill and seal the prepared solution in dry sterilized glass bottle and place the rubber closure.

6. Sterilization

Sterilize the filled and sealed glass bottles by autoclaving at 121° C for 15 minutes or any other suitable method of sterilization depending on nature of product.

7. Labelling

Label the bottles in proper manner.

8. Evaluation

The product should comply the tests and standards as specified in IP (edition 1996).

The flow diagram of IV infusion is shown in Fig. 1.

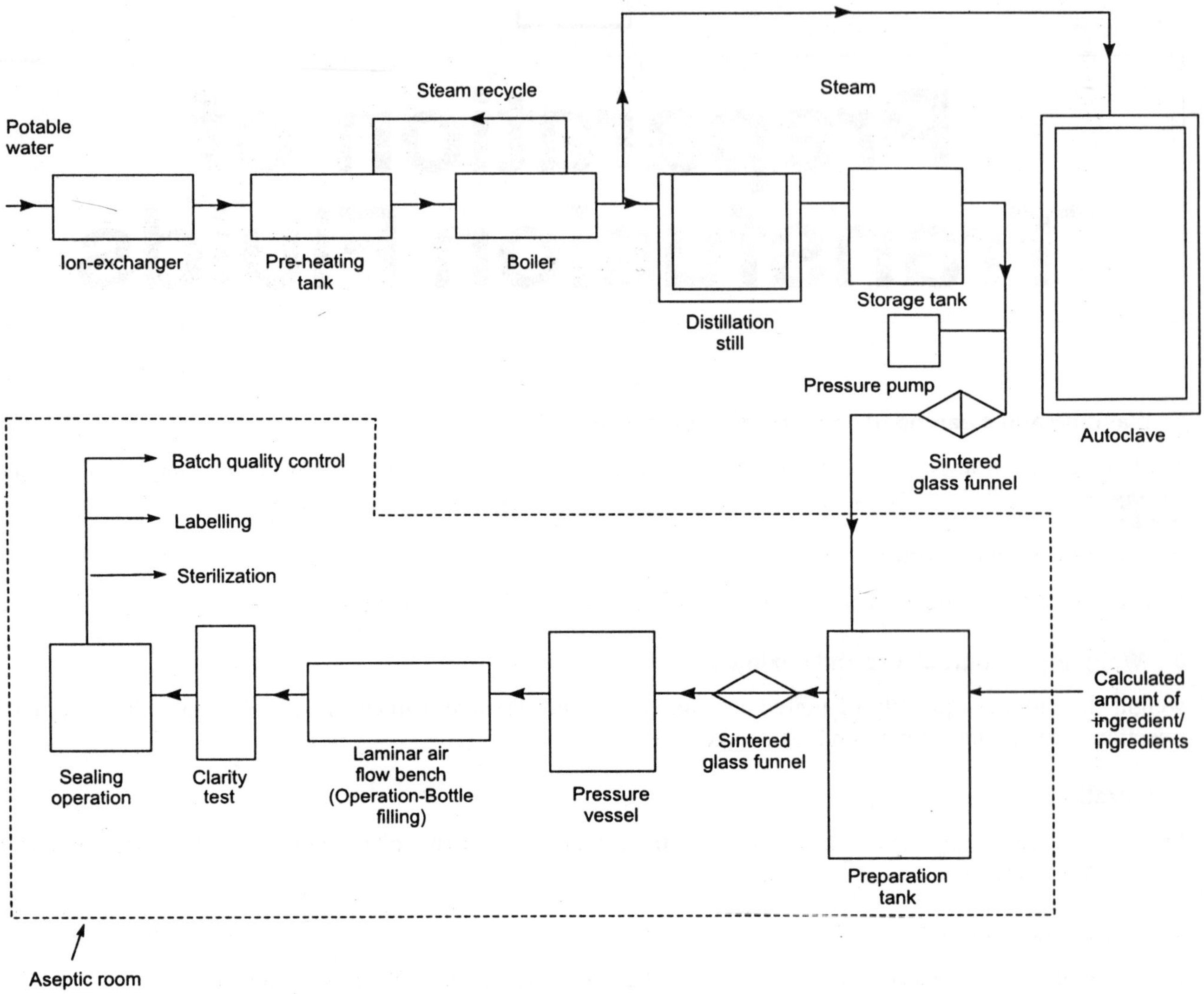

Fig. 1: Flow diagram for manufacturing (large scale) of IV infusion

Exercise 1

OBJECT

To prepare .... ml to sodium chloride injection IP (1996).

Synonym

Sodium chloride intravenous infusion.

Chemicals

Sodium chloride, water for injection.

Formula (IP)

Ingredients	*Quantity given*	*Quantity taken*
Sodium chloride	09 g	
Water for injection	q.s. 1000 ml	

Sodium chloride injection is a sterile 0.9% W/V solution of sodium chloride in water for injection. It contains no antimicrobial agent.

Procedure

(i) Wash the glass bottle and rubber closure with detergent, free flowing water followed by rinsing them with water for injection.
(ii) Sterilize the dried bottle and closure by autoclaving at 121° C for 15 minutes.
(iii) Weigh required quantity of sodium chloride and dissolve it in sufficient quantity of water for injection to make the solution up to stated volume.
(iv) Filter the above prepared solution with suitable filter media, i.e. sintered glass funnel or membrane filter or Millipore filter, etc.
(v) Fill the filtrate into dry sterilized glass bottle and place the rubber closure on glass bottle.
(vi) Sterilize the filled and sealed glass bottle by autoclaving at 121° C for 15 minutes.

Labelling

The label states

(a) the strength as the percentage W/V of sodium chloride.
(b) that a solution containing visible solid particles must not be used.

When the preparation is intended for intravenous infusion, the label states that the injection contains approximately 150 millimoles each of sodium and chloride ions per litre.

Storage

Store in single dose container of glass or plastic, in a cool place. On keeping, small solid particles may separate from a glass containers. A solution containing such particles may not be used.

Use

As electrolyte replenisher.

Exercise 2

OBJECT

To prepare .... ml of compound sodium chloride injection IP (1996).

Synonym

Ringer's injection.

Chemicals

Sodium chloride, potassium chloride, calcium chloride and water for injection.

IP Formula

Ingredients	*Quantity given*	*Quantity taken*
Sodium chloride	8.6 g	
Potassium chloride	0.3 g	
Calcium chloride	0.33 g	
Water for injection	q.s. 1000 ml	

Compound sodium chloride injection is a sterile solution containing 0.86% W/V of sodium chloride, 0.03% W/V of potassium chloride and 0.033% W/V of calcium chloride in water for injection. It contains no antimicrobial agent.

Procedure

(i) Wash the glass bottle and rubber closure with detergent, free flowing water followed by rinsing them with water for injection.
(ii) Sterilize the dried bottle and closure by autoclaving at 121° C for 15 minutes.
(iii) Weigh required quantity of sodium chloride, potassium chloride, calcium chloride and dissolve in sufficient quantity of water for injection to make the solution up to stated volume.
(iv) Filter the above prepared solution with suitable filter media, i.e. sintered glass funnel or membrane filter or millipore filter, etc.
(v) Fill the filterate into dry sterilized glass bottle and place the rubber closure on glass bottle.
(vi) Sterilize the filled and sealed glass bottle by autoclaving at 121° C for 15 minutes.

Labelling

The label states

(a) the strength as the percentage W/V of sodium chloride, potassium chloride and calcium chloride
(b) that a solution containing visible solid particles must not be used.

When the preparation is intended for intravenous infusion, the label states that the injection contains in millimoles per litre, the following approximate amount of ions; sodium,147.5; potassium,4; calcium, 2.25 and chloride, 156.

Storage

Store in single dose containers of glass or plastic. On keeping small solid particles may separate from glass containers. A solution containing such particles may not be used.

Use: As electrolyte replenisher.

Exercise 3

OBJECT

To prepare .... ml of 5% W/V dextrose injection IP (1996).

Synonyms

Dextrose intravenous infusion, Glucose intravenous infusion

Chemicals

Dextrose and water for injection

Formula IP

Ingredients	*Quantity given*	*Quantity taken*
Dextrose	05 g	
water for injection	q.s. 100 ml	

Dextrose injection is a sterile solution of dextrose in water for injection.

Procedure

(i) Wash the glass bottle and rubber closure with detergent, free flowing water followed by rinsing them with water for injection.
(ii) Sterilize the dried bottle and closure by autoclaving at 121° C for 15 minutes.
(iii) Weigh required quantity of dextrose and dissolve in sufficient quantity of water for injection to make the solution up to stated volume.
(iv) Filter the above prepared solution with suitable filter media, i.e. sintered glass funnel or membrane filter or millipore filter, etc.
(v) Fill the filterate into dry sterilized glass bottle and place the rubber closure on glass bottle.
(vi) Sterilize the filled and sealed glass bottle by autoclaving at 121° C for 15 minutes.

Labelling

The label states
(a) the strength as the percentage W/V of anhydrous dextrose, $C_6H_{12}O_6$.
(b) that a solution containing visible solid particles must not be used.

Storage

Store in single dose containers in a cool place.

Use

Nutrient and fluid replenisher.

Exercise 4

OBJECT

To prepare .... ml of sodium chloride (0.9% W/V) and dextrose (5% W/V) injection IP 1996.

Synonyms

Sodium chloride and dextrose intravenous infusion;
Sodium chloride and glucose injection;
Sodium chloride and glucose intravenous infusion.

Chemicals

Dextrose, sodium chloride, water for injection.

IP Formula

Ingredients	*Quantity given*	*Quantity taken*
Dextrose	50 g	
Sodium chloride	09 g	
Water for injection	q.s. 1000 ml	

Procedure

(i) Wash the glass bottle and rubber closure with detergent, free flowing water followed by rinsing them with water for injection.
(ii) Sterilize the dried bottle and closure by autoclaving at 121° C for 15 minutes.
(iii) Weigh required quantity of dextrose, sodium chloride and dissolve in sufficient quantity of water for injection to make the solution up to stated volume.
(iv) Filter the above prepared solution with suitable filter media, i.e. sintered glass funnel or membrane filter or millipore filter, etc.
(v) Fill the filterate into dry sterilized glass bottle and place the rubber closure on glass bottle.
(vi) Sterilize the filled and sealed glass bottle by autoclaving at 121° C for 15 minutes.

Labelling

The label states:

a. the strength as the percentage W/V of dextrose and sodium chloride.
b. that a solution containing visible solid particles must not be used.

When the preparation is intended for intravenous infusion, the label states the approximate concentration, in millimoles per litre, of sodium and chloride ions and the number of grams per litre of dextrose, $C_6H_{12}O_6$.

Storage

Store in single dose containers in a cool place, on keeping, small solid particles may separate from a glass container. A solution containing such particles may not be used.

Use

Nutrient, fluid and electrolyte replenisher.

Exercise 5

OBJECT

To prepare........................ ml of sodium lactate injection IP (1996)

Synonym

Sodium lactate intravenous infusion

Chemicals

Lactic acid, sodium hydroxide, dil. hydrochloric acid and water for injection.

Formula IP

Ingredients	*Quantity given*	*Quantity taken*
Lactic acid	12.8 ml	
Sodium hydroxide	6.6 g	
Dil. hydrochloric acid	Sufficient quantity	
water for injection	q.s. 1000 ml	

Sodium lactate injection is a sterile solution containing 1.85% W/V of sodium lactate in water for injection. It is prepared from lactic Acid with the aid of sodium hydroxide and sufficient dilute hydrochloric acid to adjust the pH of the solution.

Principle

Lactic Acid reacts with sodium hydrochloride to form sodium lactate.

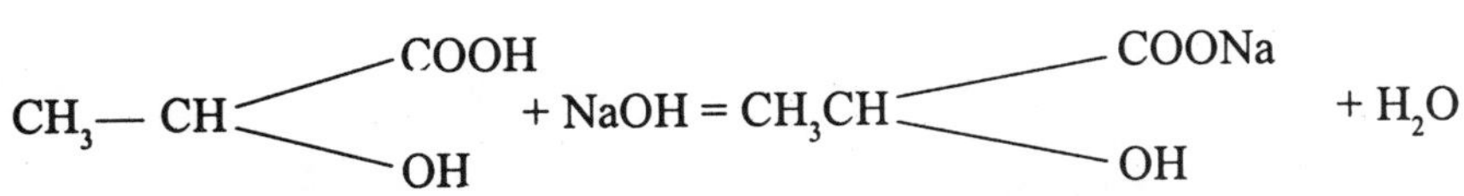

Lactic acid Sodium Lactate

The above formed lactıc acid contains a small proportion of anhydride which can be hydrolysed back to lactic acid by subjecting it to autoclaving temperature in presence of a slight excess of the alkali. The excess of alkali remaining after autoclaving is neutralised by dilute HCl.

Procedure

(i) Wash the glass bottle and rubber closure with detergent, free flowing water followed by rinsing them with water for injection.

(ii) Sterilize the dried bottle and closure by autoclaving at 121° C for 15 minutes.

(iii) Weigh the required quantity of sodium hydrochloride in to a conical flask and dissolve it in 200 ml of water for injection. Add calculated volume of lactic acid and heat in an autoclave for 1 hour. Allow the solution to

cool and add dilute hydroloride acid to adjust the pH between 5 to 7.0 using phenol red solution. Make up the stated volume with sufficient quantity of water for injection.

(iv) Filter the above prepared solution with suitable filter media, i.e. sinterd glass funnel or membrane filter or millipore filter.

(v) Fill the clear filterate in to dry sterilize glass bottle and close the bottle with rubber closure.

(vi) Sterilize the filled and sealed glass bottle by autoclaving.

Labelling

The label states:

(a) That the injection is one six molar and contains in one litre approximately 167 millimoles each of sodium ions and of bicarbonate ions (as lactate).

(b) That the injection should not be used if the solution contains visible solid particles.

Storage

Store in single dose containers of glass or plastic, in a cool place. On keeping, small solid particles may separate from the solutions in glass containers. A solution containing such particles may not be used.

pH

Between 5.0 and 7.0.

Dose

By intravenous infusion at the rate of 5 ml or less per minute.

Use

Fluid and electrolyte replenisher. Also to combat metabolic acidosis.

Exercise 6

OBJECT

To prepare .... ml of a compound sodium lactate injection (IP1996).

Synonyms

Hartmann's solution for injection.
Ringer— lactate solution for injection.

Chemicals

Lactic acid, sodium hydroxide, sodium chloride, potassium chloride, calcium chloride, Dilute hydrochloride acid, phenol red solution and water for injection.

Formula IP

Ingredients	*Quantity given*	*Quantity taken*
Lactic acid	2.4 ml	
Sodium hydroxide	1.15 g	
Dilute HCl	Sufficient quantity	
Potassium chloride	0.4 g	
Calcium chloride	0.27 g	
Water for injection	q.s. 1000 ml	

Compound sodium lactate injection is a sterile solution containing 0.24% v/v of lactic acid (equivalent to 0.32% W/V of sodium lactate) with 0.6% W/V of sodium chloride, 0.04% W/V of potassium chloride and 0.027% W/V of calcium chloride in water for injection.

Principle

Lactic acid react with sodium hydrochloride to form sodium lactate.

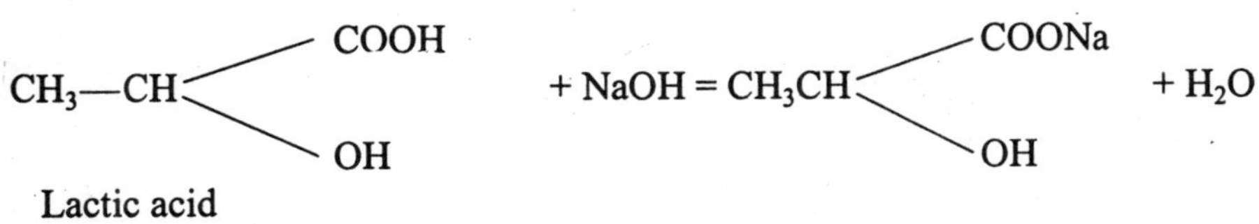

Lactic acid

Sodium lactate

The above formed lactic acid contains a small proportion of anhydride which can be hydrolysed back to lactic acid by subjecting it to autoclaving temperature in presence of a slight excess of the alkali. The excess of alkali remaining after autoclaving is neutralised by dilute HCl.

Procedure

(i) Wash the glass bottle and rubber closure with detergent, free flowing water following by rinsing them with water for injection.

(ii) Sterilize the dried bottle and closure by autoclaving at 121° C for 15 minutes.

(iii) (a) Weigh the required quantity of sodium hydroxide in to a conical flask and dissolve it in 200 ml of water for injection. Add calculated volume of lactic acid and heat in a autoclave for 1 hour. Allow the solution to cool and add dilute HCl to adjust the pH between 5 to 7 using phenol red solution (colour change red to orange).

(b) Weigh the calculated amount of sodium chloride, potassium chloride, calcium chloride and dissolve them in a sufficient quantity of water for injection in to a beaker. Mix the solution (a) and solution (b) in to a volumetric flask and make the required volume with sufficient quantity of water for injection.

(iv) Filter the above prepared solution with suitable filter media, i.e. sinterd glass funnel or membrane filter or Millipore filter.

(v) Fill the clear filtrate in to dry sterilize glass bottle and close the bottle with rubber closure.

(vi) Sterilize the filled and sealed glass bottle by autoclaving.

Labelling

The label states

(1) that the injection contains, in millimoles per litre, the following approximate amount of ions; sodium, 131, potassium, 5 calcium, 2 bicarbonate (as lactate), 29 and chloride, 111.

(2) that the injection should not be used if the solution contains visible solid particles.

Storage

Store in single dose containers of glass or plastic, in a cool place. On keeping small solid particles may separate from the solution in glass containers. A solution containing such particles may not be used.

pH

Between 5.0 to 7.0.

Use

Fluid and electrolyte replenisher.

Exercise 7

OBJECT

To prepare ....ml of 10% mannitol intravenous infusion IP (1996).

Chemicals

Mannitol, water for injection.

Formula IP

Ingredients	*Quantity given*	*Quantity taken*
Mannitol	10 g	
Water for injection	q.s. 100 ml	

Mannitol injection is a sterile solution of mannitol in water for injection.

Procedure

(i) Wash the glass bottle and rubber closure with detergent, free flowing water following by rinsing them with water for injection.
(ii) Sterilize the dries bottle and closure by autoclaving at 121° C for 15 minutes.
(iii) Weigh the required quantity of mannitol and dissolve in sufficient quantity of water for injection. Gently warm the solution if mannitol does not dissolve. Make the solution up to stated volume.
(iv) Filter the above prepared solution with suitable filter media, i.e. sinterd glass funnel or membrane filter or Millipore filter.
(v) Fill the clear filtrate in to dry sterilize glass bottle and close the bottle with rubber closure.
(vi) Sterilize the filled and sealed glass bottle by autoclaving.

Labelling

The label states
(a) the strength as a percentage W/V of mannitol
(b) that the injection should not be used if it contains visible solid particles which do not dissolve on warming.

Storage

Store at temperature between 20 and 30°. Exposure to lower temperature may cause the deposition of crystals which should be dissolved by warming before use.

Use

Osmotic diuretic.

Dose

By intravenous infusion 50 to 200 g over 24 hours but not more than 50 g on one occasion preceded by a test dose of 200 mg per kg body weight by slow intravenous injection.

Viva Voce

Q1. What is transfusion fluid ?

Ans. Large volume parenterals, intended to be administered by IV. route are called transfusion fluid.

Q2. Write uses of transfusion fluid.

Ans. 1. As electrolyte replenisher.
2. To provide nutrition.
3. In poisoning to promote diuresis.

Q3. What is isotonicity?

Ans. Isotonicity is made up of two words, i.e. *iso* means same and tonic means osmotic pressure. So solutions with same osmotic pressure are isotonic. The process of adjusting tonicity of transfusion fluid is called isotonicity. Transfusion fluid is isotonic with blood plasma.

Q4. What will happen if tonicity of solutions is not adjusted?

Ans. The solutions, which are not isotonic with plasma, may be harmful to use. When hypotonic solutions are injected in blood stream, water enters in to red blood cells and the cells swell rapidly until they burst leading to haemolysis.
When hypertonic solution is injected in to blood stream water passes outwards through the cell wall causing shrinkage (crenulation).

Q5. What is hypertonic and hypotonic solution?

Ans. Hypertonic solutions are those solutions whose osmotic pressure is higher than that of blood plasma. Hypotonic solutions are those solutions whose osmotic pressure is lower than that of blood plasma.

Q6. How will you adjust the tonicity of the transfusion fluids?

Ans. The following methods are useful for the adjustment of tonicity of transfusion fluid.
(a) Depression in freezing point and molecular concentration.
(b) Sodium chloride equivalents.

Q7. Write the formula for adjustment of tonicity of transfusion fluids by depression in freezing point and molecular concentration.

Ans. Depression in freezing point:
The temperature at which blood plasma freezes is – 0.52° C. All solutions, which freeze at–0.52° C, will be isotonic with blood plasma.

$$\text{Percentage W/V of adjusting substance required} = \frac{0.52 - x}{Y}$$

Where x = freezing point of unadjusted solution
Y = The freezing point of 1% W/V solution of the adjusting substance.

Molecular concentration

Any solution which have a molecular concentration of 0.03% will be isotonic with blood plasma.

(i) For non–ionising substance-
W/V percentage of substance required = 0.03 × g molecular weight of the substance

(ii) For ionising substance-

$$\text{W/V percentage of substance required} = \frac{0.03 \times \text{g mol. wt. of the substance}}{\text{no. of ions yielded by the substance}}$$

Q8. What are the quality controls for transfusion fluids?

Ans. (i) Sterility test.

(ii) Pyrogen test or bacterial endotoxins.

(iii) Clarity test (Particulate matter).

Q9. Why do large volume parenteral preparations (transfusion fluids) not contain any preservatives?

Ans. Since it is meant for single dose use and the contents of these remain sterile until it is injected. If preservatives are added in to transfusion fluid, they will impart toxicity in the body.

Q10. Are aseptic technique and sterilization equal?

Ans. No, aseptic technique is not a process of sterilization.

Q11. Explain aseptic technique.

Ans. It is the process of providing aseptic area, i.e. microbes free working condition during processing. Thus it prevents contamination of the product.

Q12. Give examples of aseptic techniques.

Ans. (i) Aseptic chambers or cabinet.

(ii) Laminar air flow bench.

Q13. Name the filters used in laminar air flow bench.

Ans. (i) Pre filter.

(ii) HEPA–Filter (High efficiency particulate air).

Q14. Define intravenous infusions.

Ans. Intravenous infusions are sterile aqueous solutions or emulsion with water as the continuous phase. They are free from pyrogens or bacterial endotoxins are usually made isotonic with blood and do not contain any added antimicrobial preservatives.

2

Testing of Raw Materials Used in Preparation of Transfusion Fluids

Exercise 8

OBJECTS

Testing of water for injection as raw material used in preparation of transfusion fluid.

Chemicals

Potassium chloride, alkaline potassium mercury-iodide, nitric acid, silver nitrate, diphenylamine solution, sulphuric acid, HCl, barium chloride, Potassium permanganate, methyl red, bromothymol blue.

Principle

Water for injection is non- pyrogenic distilled water intended for use in the preparation of medicines for parenteral administration. Water for injection complies with the tests described under purified water (IP) with additional requirement bacterial endotoxins as specified in Indian pharmacopeia 1996. The following tests can be performed to confirm its suitability.

Procedure

S. No.	*Tests*	*Observations*	*Inference*
1.	**Acidity or alkalinity** (a) Take 10 ml freshly boiled sample and cooled. Add 0.05 ml of methyl red solution.	(i) Solution is red (ii) Solution is not red	Does not pass Passes the test

(*Contd.*)

S. No.	*Tests*	*Observations*	*Inference*
	(b) To another 10 ml add 0.1 ml of bromothymol blue solution.	(i) Solution is blue (ii) solution is not blue	Does not pass Passes the test
2.	**Ammonium** Take two test tube, mark the no 1 and 2. In test tube no.1, take 20 ml sample, add 1 ml alkaline potassium mercury-iodide solution and allow to stand for five minutes. In test tube no. 2, take 7.5 ml of liquid being examined. Add 2.5 ml of dilute `ammonium chloride solution followed by adding 1 ml of alkaline potassium mercury-iodide solution	(i) colour of solution of test tube no.1 is not more intense than that of colour of solution of test tube no. 2 (ii) Colour of solution of test tube no.1 is more intense than that of colour of solution of test tube no.2	Passes the test Does not pass
3.	**Chloride** To 10 ml add 1 ml of 2M nitric acid, 0.2 ml of 0.1M silver nitrate. The appearance of the solution does not change for at least 15 minutes.	(i) The appearance of solution does not change for at least 15 minutes (ii) The appearance of the solution changes with in 15 minutes	Passes the test Does not pass
4.	**Sulphate** To 10 ml add 0.1 ml of 2M HCl and 0.1 ml of barium chloride solution.	(i) The appearance of the solution does not change for at least 1 hour (ii) The appearance of the solution changes	Passes the test Does not pass
5.	**Oxidisible substances** To 100 ml add 10 ml of 1M sulphuric acid and 0.1 ml of 0.02M potassium permanganate and boil for 5 minutes	(i) Solution remains faintly pink (ii) The colour of solution vanishes	Passes the test Does not pass
6.	**Nitrate** To 5 ml in a test tube immersed in ice, add 0.4 ml of a 10% W/V solution of potassium chloride, 0.1 ml of diphenylamine solution and drop wise with shaking, 5 ml of sulphuric acid. Transfer the tube to a water bath at 50° and allow to stand for 15 minutes. Prepare the standard solution in the same manner using a mixture of 4.5 ml of nitrogen free water and 0.5 ml of nitrate standard solution (2 ppm NO_3).	(i) Blue colour of test solution is not intense than that of standard solution (ii) Blue colour of test solution is intense than that of standard solution	Passes the test Does not pass

Result

Acidity or alkalinity	–	Passes/does not pass
Ammonium	–	Passes/does not pass
Chloride	–	Passes/does not pass
Sulphate	–	Passes/does not pass
Oxidisible substances	–	Passes/does not pass
Nitrate	–	Passes/does not pass

Reagents

Potassium mercury-iodide solution, alkaline

To 3.5 g of potassium iodide add 1.25 g of mercuric chloride dissolve in 80 ml of water, add a cold saturated solution of mercuric chloride in water with constant stirring until a slight red precipitate. remains. Dissolve 12 g of sodium hydroxide in the solution, add a little more of the cold saturated solution of mercuric chloride and sufficient water to produce 100 ml. Allow to stand and decant the clear supernatant liquid.

Silver nitrate 0.1M

Dissolve 17 g in sufficient water to produce 1000 ml. Standardize the solution.

Nitrate standard solution (2 ppm)

Dilute 1 volume of nitrate standard solution (100 ppm) to 50 volume with water.

Nitrate standard solution (100 ppm)

Dilute 1 volume of a 0.163% W/V solution of potassium nitrate to 10 volumes with water.

Potassium per magnate (0.02M)

Dissolve 3.2 g of potassium per magnate in 1000 ml of water, heat on a water bath for 1 hour, allow to stand for two days and filter through glass wool. The solution must be standardized.

Nitric acid xM

Solution of any molarity xM may be prepared by diluting 63x ml of nitric acid to 1000 ml with water.

HCl xM

Solution of any molarity xM may be prepared by diluting 85x ml of HCl to 1000 ml with water.

Diphenylamine solution

0.1% W/V solution of diphenylamine in sulphuric acid.

Barium chloride solution

10% W/V solution of barium chloride.

Sulphuric acid xM

Solution of any molarity xM may be prepared by carefully adding 54x ml of sulphuric acid to an equal volume of water and diluting to 1000 ml with water.

Exercise 9

OBJECT

Testing of dextrose as raw material used in preparation of transfusion fluid.

Chemicals

phenolphthalein, chloride standard solution (125 ppm), sulphate standard solution (200 ppm), sodium hydroxide, barium chloride, acetic acid, sulphuric acid.

Principle

Dextrose is D(+) glucopyranose which is available in two form, i.e. dextrose anhydrous and dextrose monohydrate. Anhydrous form of dextrose is used in preparation of transfusion fluid. Indian pharmacopoeia includes various standards. The sample of dextrose should not be of pharmacopoeial quality unless it complies with all the requirements stated, i.e. acidity or alkalinity, clarity, colour and odour of solution, specific optical rotation, arsenic, heavy metals, chloride, sulphate, barium, foreign sugars, soluble starch and dextrins, sulphated ash, water, pyrogens.

Procedure

S. No.	*Tests*	*Observations*	*Reference*
1.	**Acidity or alkalinity** Dissolve 6 g in 25 ml of carbon dioxide free water and add 0.3 ml phenolphthalein solution. The solutionis colourless and not more than 0.15 ml of 0.1M sodium hydroxide is required to change the colour of solution to pink.	on addition of phenolphthalein, the resulting solution should be colourless. On adding 0.15 ml of 0.1M NaOH, the colour of solution should change to pink.	Passes the test
2.	**Chloride** Make 20 ml of 10% W/V solution of dextrose and transfer to a Nessler's cylinder. Add 10 ml of dil nitric acid, dilute to 50 ml with water and add 1 ml of 0.1M silver nitrate. Stir and allow to stand for 5 minutes protected from light. In another N. cylinder take 10 ml of standard chloride solution (125 ppm) and 5 ml of water in the same manner	1. opalescence of test solution is not more intense than that of standard solution. 2. opalescence of test solution is more intense than that of standard solution	Passes the test Does not pass
3.	**Sulphate** Take 7.5 ml of 10% W/V of a dextrose, dilute to 15 ml with distilled water, transfer it in N.cylinder, add 1 ml of 25.0% W/V solution barium chloride and 1.5 ml of ethanolic sulphate standard solution (200 ppm). Mix and allow to stand for 1 minute,	1. opalescence of test solution is not more intense than that of standard solution 2. Opalescence of test Solution is more intense than that of standard	Passes the test Does not pass the test

(*Contd.*)

S. No.	*Tests*	*Observations*	*Reference*
	add 0.15 ml of 5M acetic acid. Add water q.s. to make 50 ml Stir and allow to stand for 5 minutes. In another N. cylinder treat in the same manner 15 ml of sulphate standard solution (200 ppm) in the place of the solution being examined.	solution	
4.	**Barium** (a) Take 10 ml of 10% W/V solution of dextrose, add 1 ml of 1M sulphuric acid. Examine exactly after 1 hour. (b) In another test tube take 10 ml of 10% W/V solution of dextrose and 1 ml of water.	(i) Opalescence of solution (a) is not more intense than that of solution (b) (ii) Opalescence of solution- (a) is more intense than that of solution -(b)	Passes the test Does not pass
5.	**Foreign sugars, soluble starch and dextrins** Boil 1 g sample in 30 ml of ethanol (90%) to dissolve.	(i) The appearance of the solution does not change on cooling (ii) The appearance of solution changes on cooling.	Passes the test Does not pass

Result

Acidity or alkalinity	–	Passes/does not pass
Chloride	–	passes/does not pass
Sulphate	–	passes/does not pass
Barium	–	passes/does not pass
Foreign sugars, soluble starch and dextrins	–	passes/does not pass

Reagents

Chloride

(125 ppm)–Dilute 25 volumes of a 0.0824% W/V solution of sodium chloride to 100 volumes with water.

Sulphate standard solution (200 ppm)

Dilute 20 volumes of 0.181% W/V solution of potassium sulphate in distilled water to 100 volumes.

Sulphate standard solution 200 ppm, ethanolic

Dilute 20 volumes 0.181% W/V of solution of potassium sulphate in ethanol (30%) to 100 volumes.

Sodium hydroxide (0.1M)

Dissolve 4.2 g of sodium hydroxide in sufficient CO_2 free water to produce 1000 ml. Standardize the solution.

Sulphuric acid *x*M

Solution any molarity may be prepared by carefully adding 54x ml of sulphuric acid to a equal volume of water and diluting to 1000 ml with water.

Acetic acid *x*M

Solution of any molarity xM may be prepared by diluting 57x ml of glacial acetic acid to 1000 ml with water.

Exercise 10

OBJECT

Testing of dextrose as raw water for its water contents by Karl Fisher apparatus.

Chemicals

Karl Fisher reagent, dehydrated methanol, sodium tartrate.

Principle

Pharmacopoeia includes test for water content for dextrose (anhydrous and monohydrate form) which states that it should not more than 1% W/V (anhydrous form) and between 7% and 9.5% W/V (monohydrate).

For determination of small amount of water, Karl Fisher (1935) proposed a reagent prepared by the action of sulphur dioxide upon iodine dissolved in pyridine and methanol. Titrimetric determination of water is based upon the quantitative reaction of water with an anhydrous solution of sulphur dioxide and iodine in a presence of buffer.

% of moisture content =

$$\frac{\text{Volume of Karl Fisher reagent used} \times \text{water equivalence factor}}{\text{weight of sample in mg}}$$

KF Apparatus

The various automatic and manual apparatus is available in the market. The instrument consists of two separate unit, i.e. control unit and titration unit.

Control unit

It has been designed with latest technology which consist of on/off/ end point indicator, detector (current sending by electronic control) and timer with buzzer. Here titration is controlled automatically.

Titration unit

It consists air tight glass vessel, KF flow device, burette (10 ml capacity) and magnetic stirrer.

Procedure

1. Unless otherwise directed add about 20 ml of dehydrated methanol in the titration vessel of KF apparatus
2. Fill the auto burette up to zero mark. Switch on the KF titrimeter.
3. Remove the moisture content of methanol by titrating to the electrometric end point with the KF reagent.
4. Transfer quickly the prescribed amount of the substance being examined accurately weighed in to the titration vessel.
5. Titrate again till electrometric end point is reached.
6. Take the final reading of the burette and find out the quantity of KF reagent used. Calculate the percentage of moisture content of the sample.

Result

The given sample (dextrose anhydrous) passes/does not pass the test for water content (IP limit is not more than 1.0% W/W).

Exercise 11

OBJECT

Testing of sodium chloride as raw material used in preparation of transfusion fluid.

Chemicals

Bromothymol blue, HCl, NaOH, Dil H_2SO_4, phenol red, sodium thiosulphate, KBr, ferric ammonium sulphate, sodium nitrite, Starch solution, chloramines solution.

Principle

Sodium chloride is widely used in preparation of transfusion fluid as tonicity agent, fluid and electrolyte replenisher. The sample of sodium chloride should not be of pharmacopoeial quality unless it complies with all the requirements stated, i.e. Acidity or alkalinity; clarity and colour of the solution, arsenic, barium, bromide, calcium and magnesium, ferro cyanide, heavy metals, iodide, iron, loss on drying and potassium.

Procedure

S. No.	*Tests*	*Observations*	*Inference*
1.	**Acidity or alkalinity** Prepare 20% W/V solution of sodium chloride in carbon dioxide free water prepared from distilled water (solution A). To 20 ml of solution A, Add 0.1 ml of bromothymol blue solution	(i) Not more than 0.5 ml of 0.01M HCl or 0.01M NaOH is required to change the colour of the solution (ii) Vice versa	Passes the test Does not pass
2.	**Clarity and colour of solution** Examine the clarity and colour of the solution A	(i) Clarity and colour of the solution is same than that of water (colourless as water) (ii) Vice versa	Passes the test Does not pass the test
3.	**Barium** Dissolve 2 g in 10 ml of water, and add 2 ml of dilute sulphuric acid	(i) No turbidity is produced (ii) Turbidity is produced	Passes the test Does not pass the test
4.	**Bromide** (A) Dissolve 1 g in sufficient water to produce 100 ml to 0.5 ml of solution, add 9 ml of water, 1 ml of phenol red solution and 0.05 ml of chloramine solution. Shake for 15 seconds and add 0.15 ml of 0.1M sodium thiosulphate.	(i) Violet colour of solution A is not intense than that of solution B (ii) Violet colour of solution A is intense than that of solution B	Passes the test Does not pass the test

(*Contd.*)

S. No.	Tests	Observations	Inference
	(B) Solution is prepared at the same time and in same manner using 0.5 ml of 0.0015% W/V solution of KBr and 9 ml of water		
5.	**Ferro cyanide** Dissolve 2 g in 6 ml of water and add 0.5 ml of mixture of 5 ml of 1% W/V solution of ferric ammonium sulphate in a 0.25% W/V solution of sulphuric acid, and 95 ml of 1% W/V solution of ferrous sulphate.	(i) No blue colour is produced within 10 minutes (ii) Blue colour is produced within 10 minutes	Passes the test Does not pass the test
6.	**Iodide** Moisten 5 g by adding drop wise a solution freshly prepared by mixing 25 ml of iodide free starch solution, 2 ml of 0.5 ml sulphuric acid, 0.5 ml of sodium nitrite solution and 25 ml of water	(i) Blue colour is not being shown after 5 minutes (ii) Blue colour is shown after 5 minutes	Passes the test Does not pass the test

Result

Acidity and alkalinity	–	Passes/does not pass
Clarity and colour the solution	–	Passes/does not pass
Barium	–	Passes/does not pass
Bromide	–	Passes/does not pass
Ferrocyanide	–	Passes/does not pass
Iodide	–	Passes/does not pass

Reagents

1. Chloramine solution

2.0% W/V solution of chloramine. Prepare immediately before use.

2. Sodium nitrite solution

10% W/V solution of sodium nitrite. Prepare immediately before use.

3. Starch solution

Triturate 1 g of soluble starch with 5 ml of water and add, stirring continuously to 100 ml of boiling water. Prepare immediately before use.

4. Sodium thiosulphate 0.1M

Dissolve 25 g of sodium thiosulphate and 0.2 g of sodium carbonate in carbon dioxide free water and dilute to 1000 ml with the same solvent. Standardize the solution.

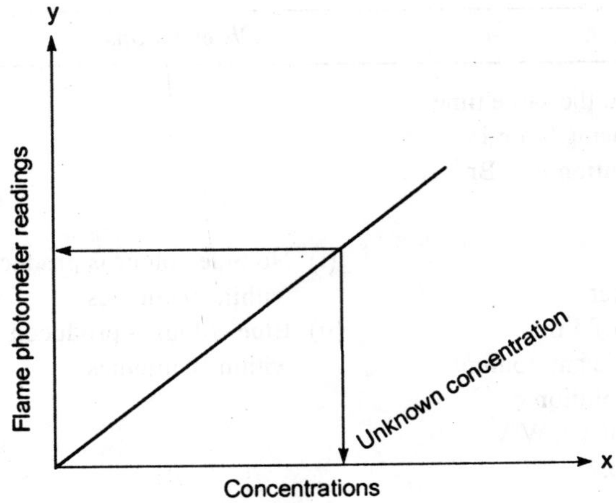
y
x
Flame photometer readings
Concentrations
Unknown concentration

Fig. 2

Exercise 12

OBJECT

Estimation of potassium in given sample of sodium chloride as raw material used in preparation of transfusion fluid.

Chemicals

Potassium chloride, distilled water.

Principle

Indian pharmacopoeia states, the sodium chloride intended for use in the manufacture of injectable preparations should not contain more than 0.1% of potassium, determined by flame photometry.

The operation of flame photometer is based on characteristic emissions of the elements when their fluids under analysis is sprayed as a fine mist into a non luminous flame. The detector views the flame through a narrow band optical filter. The output of the detector is connected to on electronic metering unit which provides digital readouts. Before analysing the unknown fluids the system is standardized with solution of known concentration of elements under examination.

Procedure

Prepare a series of standard solution. Select the 768 nm wavelength filter. Feed distilled water to the atomizer to set zero read out. Spray the most concentrated standard solution in to the flame and set to full scale deflection/ digital read out. Again spray distilled water in to the flame and read just it to zero. Spray each standard solution in to the flame three times and record the readings. Wash the apparatus thoroughly with water. After each spraying plot the standard curve between the mean of each group of three readings against the concentration. Take the reading by spraying the sample solution (1% W/V). Find out the concentration of potassium per ml in the sample and calculate potassium (percentage) in given sample of sodium chloride.

Result

Passes/does not pass.

Reagents

Sodium Chloride Solution

1.0% W/V dissolve 1 g of sodium Chloride in sufficient quantity of distilled water to produce the volume 100 ml.

Potassium solution standard stock solution

Dissolve 1.1440 g of potassium chloride, previously dried to constant weight at 130° C in sufficient freshly distilled water to produce 1000 ml potassium solution contains 600 μg of potassium in per ml.

Take the above standard stock solution as per given table and dilute to 100 ml with distilled water.

Stock solution		*Concentration in μg/ml*
10 ml	–	60 μg/ml
20 ml	–	120 μg/ml
40 ml	–	240 μg/ml
80 ml	–	480 μg/ml

Note

Indian pharmacopoeia 1996 states, several instruments (Flame photometer) of suitable selectivity are available. The manufacturer's instructions for the operation of the instrument should be strictly followed.

Electronic metering unit which provides digital readouts. By calibrating this instrument with standard solutions, one can find out the concentration of unknown sample without plotting the standard curve.

Exercise 13

OBJECT

Testing of mannitol as raw material used in preparation of transfusion fluid.

Chemicals

Phenolphthalein, HCl, NaOH, silver nitrate, acetic acid, barium chloride.

Principle

The sample of mannitol should not be of pharmacopoeial quality unless it complies with all the requirements stated, i.e. acidity or alkalinity clarity and colour of solution, specific optical rotation, arsenic; chloride; sulphate; reducing sugar; sorbitol; sulphated ash; loss on drying; pyrogens.

Procedure

S. No.	*Tests*	*Observations*	*Inference*
1.	**Acidity or alkalinity** Dissolve 0.5 g of sample in sufficient CO_2 free water prepared from distilled water (solution A) to 5 ml of solution A add 5 ml of CO_2 free water and 0.05 ml of dilute phenolphthalein solution. To further 5 ml of solution A, Add 5 ml of CO_2 free water and 0.05 ml methyl red solution.	(i) Not more than 0.2 ml of 0.01M sodium hydroxide is required to change the colour of the solution to pink. Not more than 0.3 ml of 0.01M HCl is required to change the colour of the solution to red	Passes the test
		(ii) More than the stated volume of NaOH and HCl is required to change the colour of the solution.	Does not pass
2.	**Clarity and colour of solution** Examine the clarity and colour of the solution A.	(i) Clarity and colour is same than that of water (colourless as water)	Passes the test
		(ii) vice versa	Does not pass
3.	**Chloride** A solution of 0.5 g in 10 ml of water transfer to a Nessler cylinder. Add 10 ml dilute nitric. acid, dilute to 50 ml with water and add 1 ml of 0.1M silver nitrate. Stir and allow to stand for 5 minutes	(i) Opalescence of test solution is not more intense than that of standard solution	Passes the test
		(ii) Opalescence of test solution is more intense than that	Does not pass

(Contd.)

S. No.	*Tests*	*Observations*	*Inference*
	protected from light. In another Nessler cylinder, take 10 ml of chloride standard solution (50 ppm) and 5 ml of water in the same manner.	of standard solution.	
4.	**Sulphate** A solution of 1.5 g in 10 ml of water, dilute to 15 ml with distilled water, transfer it in Nessler cylinder, add 1 ml 25.0% W/V solution of barium chloride and 0.5 ml of ethanolic sulphate standard solution (100 ppm). Mix and allow to stand for 1 minute, add 0.15 ml 5M acetic acid. Add water q.s. to make 50 ml. Stir and allow to stand for 5 minutes. In another nessler cylinder treat in the same manner taking 15 ml of sulphate standard solution (100 ppm) in the place of the solution being examined.	(i) Opalescence of the test solution is not more intense than that of the colour standard solution	Passes the test
		(ii) Opalescence of test solution is more intense than that of the colour of standard solution.	Does not pass

Result

Acidity or alkalinity	–	Passes/does not pass
Clarity and colour of solution	–	Passes/does not pass
Chloride	–	Passes/does not pass
Sulphate	–	Passes/does not pass

Reagents

Acetic acid *x*M

Solution of any molarity may be prepared by diluting 57*x* ml of glacial acetic acid to 1000 ml with water.

Silver nitrate *x*M

Solution of any molarity *x*M may be prepared by dissolving 170 x g of silver nitrate in sufficient water to produce 1000 ml store in light resistant container.

Chloride standard solution–50 ppm

Dilute 10 volumes of a 0.0824% W/V solution of sodium chloride to 100 volumes with water.

Sulphate standard solution 100 ppm

Dilute 10 volumes of a 0.181% W/V solution of potassium sulphate in distilled water to 100 volumes with the same solvent.

Sulphate standard solution 100 ppm ethanolic

Dilute 10 volumes of a 0.181% W/V solution of potassium sulphate in ethanol (30%) to 100 volumes with ethanol (30%).

Exercise 14

OBJECT

To carry out hydrolytic test on glass bottles used for manufacturing of transfusion fluid.

Chemicals

Methyl red solution, 0.01M HCl.

Principle

Hydrolytic resistance is the resistance to release alkaline ions into attacking media under the conditions specified from interior surface of the container. The degree of attack is determined by the amount of alkalinity released from the glass. This quantity of alkali is extremely small in the case of more resistance glass (Type I or II glass).

The Indian pharmacopoeia 1996 states the following limit for glass bottle used in transfusion fluid.

Capacity of container (corresponding to 90% average overflow volume in ml)	Volume of 0.01M HCl per 100 ml of test solution type I or II glass (ml)
More than 200 but not more than 500	0.30
More than 500	0.20

Procedure

Take at least three unused glass bottles. Rinse each container at least twice with water at room temperature and finally with fresh distilled water. Fill the containers to brim with freshly prepared distilled water, empty them and determine the average overflow volume. Fill the bottles to 90% their calculated overflow volume and cover them with borosilicate glass dishes or aluminium foil previously rinsed with fresh distilled water. Place the containers in an autoclave. Switch on the autoclave. Raise the temperature from 100 to 121° over 20 minutes. Maintain the temperature of 121° for 60 minutes and reduce the temperature from 121 to 100° over 40 minutes. Remove the containers from autoclave and cool them in running water. Combine the liquid from containers being examined. Take 100 ml of above liquid in conical flask, add 0.3 ml methyl red and titrate it with 0.01 M HCl. Repeat the operation using the same volume of freshly prepared distilled water.

The difference between the two titration represents to volume of 0.01 M HCl required by the test solution.

Result

The transfusion glass bottles pass the test (hydrolytic resistance)/do not pass.

(IP limit for capacity of glass bottle 200 ml to 500 ml should not require more them 0.3 ml of 0.01M HCl).

Viva Voce

Q1. Write the application of flame photometer.

Ans. Flame photometer is capable of estimating the amount of Na, K, Ca, and lithium in given unknown sample.

Q2. Write the application of K. F. apparatus.

Ans. K.F. method for determination of moisture content is used in a large number of industries such as pharmaceutical and drug manufacturing industries, food stuff, sugar, wood, paper and textile industries, petroleum refineries, chemical fertilizer units, etc.

Q3. What is potable water?

Ans. Potable water is used for drinking purposes which is generally obtained from natural sources like well, lake, spring and river, etc.

Q4. What is purified water?

Ans. It is water which is obtained by the process of distillation, ion exchange treatment or reverse osmosis. This water is suitable for pharmaceutical uses.

Q5. What is water for injection?

Ans. It is non- pyrogenic distilled water which is obtained by distilling the potable water or purified water with an effective device for preventing the entrainment of droplets. It complies with standards described under purified water with additional test for bacterial endotoxins.

Q6. What is sterile water for injection?

Ans. It is water for injection distributed in suitable containers of glass or any other material, sealed and sterilized by heat under condition that ensure that water remains apyrogenic.

Q7. What are different type of glass used as container for pharmaceutical use?

Ans. There are three types of glass.

(A) Type–I glass—It is neutral glass (borosilicate) possesses a high hydrolytic resistance.

(B) Type–II glass—It also has a high hydrolytic resistance due to an appropriate surface treatment.

(C) Type–III glass—It offers only a moderate hydrolytic resistance. It is soda-lime silica glass.

Q8. Why type I and type II glasses are used for preparations of different types of injectable.

Ans. Because type I and type II glasses have a high hydrolytic resistance. Estimation of hydrolytic resistance test is official in IP

Q9. Write the limitation of glass container for transfusion fluid.

Ans.
(i) Weight is respectively high.
(ii) It needs rubber closures.
(iii) It is fragile.

Q10. Write advantages of plastic as containers for parenteral use.

Ans.
(i) It is lighter and cheaper than glass.
(ii) Its fabrication is easy.
(iii) It is unbreakable.

Q11. Why should water for injection be used immediately for preparation of transfusion fluid?

Ans. Because during storage the microorganisms in water may produce pyrogens.

Q12. Deionised water is preferred in boiler or water still why?

Ans. Potable water promotes scales formation. High content of chloride gives rise to corrosion of steel. Cleaning of steel or boiler is a great problem. So deionised water is preferred.

Q13. Why anhydrous form of dextrose is used in preparation of transfusion fluid?

Ans. Since monohydrate form is not pure for preparation of transfusion fluid. When its solutions will be subjected to autoclaving becomes brown colour due to carmelisation.

Q14. Why sodium lactate is used as a substitute for sodium bicarbonate?

Ans. Since sodium lactate is metabolized in the body to sodium bicarbonate.

Q15. Why pH is adjusted (pH 5 to 7) in preparation of compound sodium lactate injection IP?

Ans. Lactic acid reacts with NaOH to form sodium lactate and small proportion of anhydride which is hydrolysed back to lactic acid by subjecting to it autoclaving temperature in presence of slight excess of the alkali. The excess of alkali remains after autoclaving is neutralized by dilute HCl.

Q16. What is pyrogen?

Ans. Pyrogens are the metabolic products of microorganisms. They are soluble, filterable, thermostable and nonvolatile substances.

Q17. How are pyrogens removed?

Ans.
(i) Heating in hot air oven at a temperature of 175° C for 3–4 hours.
(ii) It can be removed by heating in a autoclave in presence of an acid, alkali or oxidizing agent.
(iii) It can be removed by adsorbing by using adsorbing agents like activated charcoal, asbestos pads or aluminium hydroxide gel.

3

Sterilization of Surgical Instruments, Glassware and other Hospital Supplies

Exercise 15

OBJECT

Sterilization of surgical instruments by dry heat method (hot air oven).

Apparatus

Surgical instruments, detergent and hot air oven.

Principle

Dry heat sterilization causes killing of microorganism and bacterial spores by oxidation. In this process, the high temperature and longer period of exposure are needed. Hot air oven is commonly used for dry heat sterilization which is electrically heated and thermostatically controlled. Heat is transferred from the source to the articles by continuous forced circulation through blower (fan), Conduction along the shelves on which the articles are placed and radiation from heated wall of oven. The Indian pharmacopoeia states the following combination of temperature and time.

Temperature (°C)	*Minimum holding time*
180°	Not less than 30 minutes.
170°	Not less than 1 hour.
160°	Not less than 2 hours.

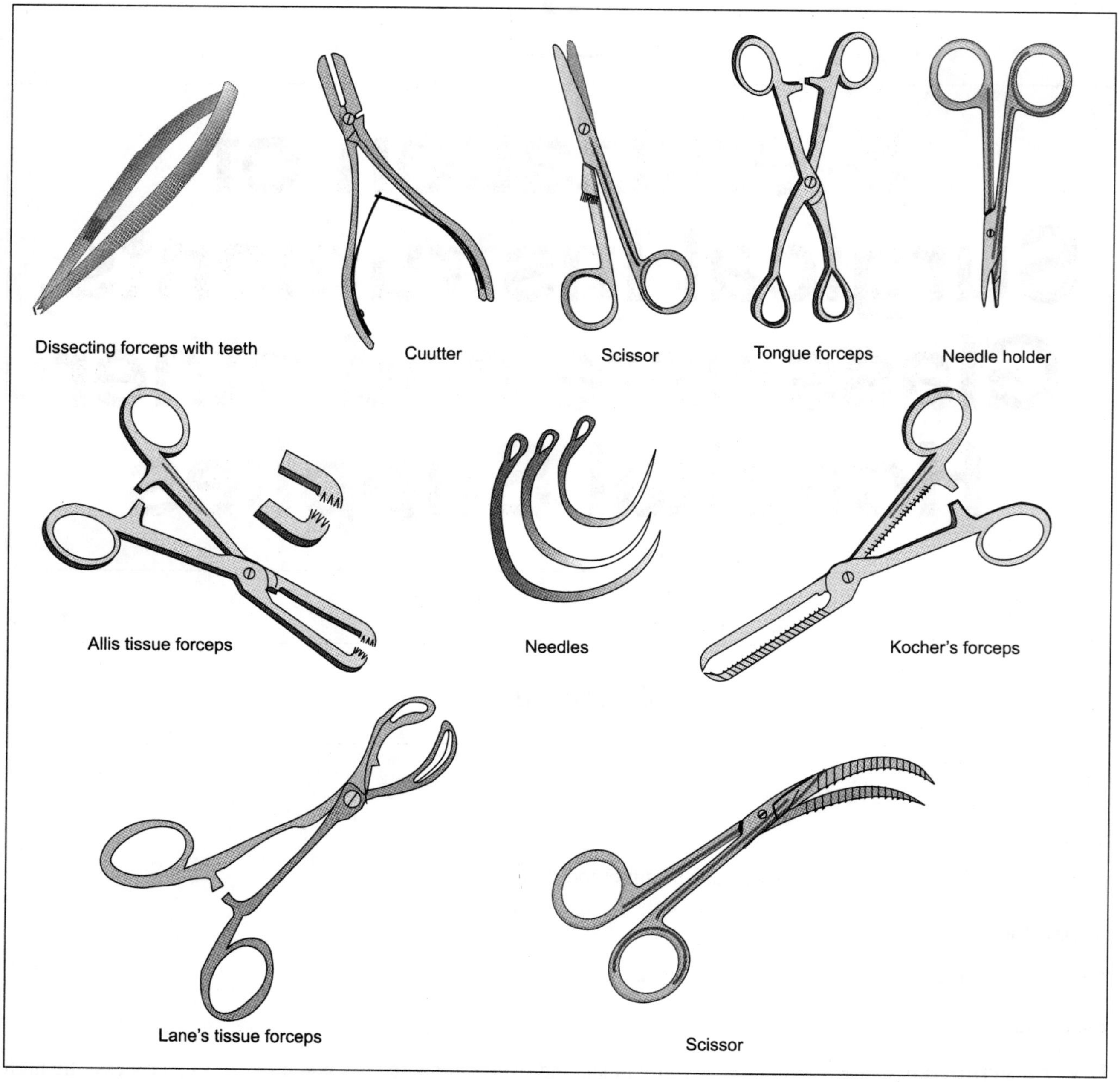
Dissecting forceps with teeth
Cuutter
Scissor
Tongue forceps
Needle holder
Allis tissue forceps
Needles
Kocher's forceps
Lane's tissue forceps
Scissor

Fig. 3:

Procedure

1. Washing of instruments

Wash the instruments with detergent water, free flowing water followed by rising with distilled water and dry them.

2. Wrapping

Wrapping of each instruments with paper of suitable thickness is needed to maintain their sterility during the cooling period.

3. Loading

The proper loading is the greatest importance. Keep the sufficient space between the instruments to allow the easy circulation of air and radiation from the wall of the oven.

4. Operation

Switch on the oven and go on heating till get the required temperature for sterilization (lag time). The condition is maintained for the required holding time (160° for two hours).

5. Cooling time

Switch off the oven and allow the oven to cool. During the cooling time the door of the oven should be kept closed. The sterilized instruments may be used immediately or may be stored.

Exercise 16

OBJECT

Sterilization of glassware by hot air oven.

Apparatus

Glassware, i.e. test tube, conical flask, beaker, petri dishes, measuring cylinder etc; paper, detergent, chromic acid mixture, hot air oven.

Principle

Dry heat sterilization causes killing of microorganism and bacterial spores by oxidation. In this process, the high temperature and longer period of exposure are needed. Hot air oven is commonly used for dry heat sterilization which is electrically heated and thermostatically controlled. Heat is transferred from the source to the articles by continuous forced circulation through blower (fan), Conduction along the shelves on which the articles are placed and radiation from heated wall of oven. The Indian pharmacopoeia states the following combination of temperature and time.

Temperature (°C)	*Minimum holding time*
180°	Not less than 30 minutes
170°	Not less than 1 hour
160°	Not less than 2 hours

Procedure

1. Washing of glassware

Wash the glassware either with chromic acid mixture or detergent solution followed by washing with free flowing water and finally prolong rinsing them with purified water.

2. Wrapping

Cover the open end test tube and conical flask with cotton wool and wrap with aluminium metal foil or paper to maintain their sterility during the cooling of the oven.

3. Loading

The proper loading is the greatest importance. Keep the sufficient space between the instruments to allow the easy circulation of air and radiation from the wall of the oven.

4. Operation

Switch on the oven and go on heating till get the required temperature for sterilization (lag time). The condition is maintained for the required holding time (160° for two hours).

5. Cooling time

Switch off the oven and allow the oven to cool. During the cooling time the door of the oven should be kept closed to avoid breakage.

The sterilized glassware may be used immediately or may be stored.

Exercise 17

OBJECT

Sterilization of surgical dressings, glassware, surgical instruments, etc. by autoclaving method.

Apparatus

Sterilizing materials, autoclave, muslin cloth and paper.

Principle

Autoclaving involves heating in an autoclave with saturated steam under pressure which causes coagulation of cell protein leading to killing of microorganisms. The thermal capacity of steam is much greater than that of hot air. The penetration power of steam is much more than that of dry heat. The Indian pharmacopoeia states the following combinations of temperature and time.

Holding temperature (°C)	*Minimum holding time in minutes*
115 to 118	30
121 to 124	15
126 to 129	10
134 to 138	03

When surgical materials are sterilized in an autoclave the steam used should neither be super heated nor contain more than 5% of entrained moisture. The most dressings are conveniently sterilized by maintaining at a temperature of 134 to 138° for 3 minutes but other suitable combinations of temperature and time may be used.

Procedure

1. Washing and packing of articles

The articles (glassware or surgical instruments) to be sterilized should be properly washed with detergent solution, free flowing water and finally rinsing with purified water. Surgical dressings to be sterilized should be formed package of required size. Wrap the package in one or two layers of paper followed by layer or layers of muslin cloth.

2. Loading

The loading must be carefully arrange in the autoclave so that space is left between the articles to allow the maximum penetration of steam. Close the lid and tighten the clamping screws. Switch on the heat source.

3. Removal of air

Keep open the air vent. After some times water of the autoclave will start boiling and steam will be generated which will replace the entire air from the body of autoclave.

4. Heating up time

Close the vent valve and let the internal pressure rise. Maintain the pressure for required time.

5. Cooling down period

Switch off the heat source and left the pressure be reached to zero. Open the air vent and lid to take out the sterilized articles. The sterilized articles may be used immediately or may be stored in a proper manner.

Reagent

Chromic acid mixture (for cleaning glassware)

Dissolve 200 g of sodium dichromate in about 100 ml of water, cooling in an ice- bath and adding slowly to it, with stirring, 1500 ml of sulphuric acid. The mixture should be prepared in borosilicate glass beaker. This mixture is extremely corrosive and hygroscopic, and should be stored in glass stoppered bottle in a safe place. When the mixture acquires a green colour, it should be discarded.

Viva Voce

Q1. Define sterilization.

Ans. Sterilization is the process by which all viable forms of microorganisms including their spores are removed or killed from preparations or articles.

Q2. Enlist the different methods of sterilization.

Ans. (i) Physical method
- (a) Dry heat sterilization
- (b) Moist heat sterilization
- (c) Sterilization by radiation

(ii) Chemical sterilization
- (a) Gaseous sterilization
- (b) sterilization by disinfectants

(iii) Mechanical method

Q3. Define D-value (decimal reduction time).

Ans. This the time in minutes required to reduce the number of viable organisms by 90%.

Q4. What is microbial survival probability of sterilized articles or preparations as per IP norms.

Ans. This value is 10^{-6}, i.e. assurance of less than one chance in one million that viable microorganisms are present in the sterilized articles or preparations.

Q5. Define Z value.

Ans. The change in temperature required to alter the D-value by factor of 10.

Q6. What is wet and dry steam?

Ans. *Wet steam:* Steam produced from a boiler contains a large number of entrained droplets of water.
Dry steam: Steam free from water droplets is referred to dry steam.

Q7. Why wet steam is not suitable for sterilization of surgical dressings?

Ans. It will reduce condensation of water vapour so that less latent heat will be made available. Since surgical dressings and paper wrappings are absorptive, they will become sodden.

Q8. Why paper packing or wrapping of articles being sterilized is essential in sterilization by hot air oven?

Ans. During the cooling period, non-sterile air may enter in to oven, so articles must be wrapped in paper or placed in metal boxes or as in the case of test tubes plugged with cotton wool or closed with aluminium caps.

Q9. Sterilization of surgical dressings is not carried out by dry heat method. Why?

Ans. Because the natural moisture of the fibres quickly vaporizes which leads to deterioration and charring of the dressings.

Q10. Write name of articles/pharmaceuticals which are sterilized by dry heat method.

Ans. Dry powder like talc, starch, lactose, etc.; minerals oil, waxes, glassware, surgical instrument, glass syringes.

Q11. Write the name of articles which are effectively sterilized by moist heat (autoclaving).

Ans. Sealed ampoules, transfusion bottles, glassware, surgical dressings, rubber gloves, surgical instruments, surgical gowns, rubber closures, etc.

Q13. Write the name of source of gamma radiation which is used in sterilization process.

Ans. Radioactive metals like cobalt –60; cesium–137.

Q14. Moist heat sterilization is not suitable for oily and fatty preparations. Why?

Ans. Because steam can not penetrate oil and fat.

Q15. What is cold sterilization?

Ans. Sterilization by radiation is cold sterilization because no heat is used in this methods.

Q16. Enlist the filters used for sterilizing the solutions by filtration.

Ans. Seitz filters, sintered glass filters, berkefed filters, millipore filters, membrane filters, etc.

Q17. How will you sterilized the surgical suture?

Ans. By gamma radiation.

Q18. The repeated sterilization of surgical dressing is not preferred why?

Ans. The repeated sterilization of surgical dressing may cause irreversible changes in the materials used in the preparation.

Q19. What is biological indicators?

Ans. It is characterized and standardized preparation of specific microorganisms having known stable high resistance to one or more sterilization processes.

Q20. What is the use of biological indicators?

Ans.
1. It helps in validity of the physical operation of a sterilizer.
2. Monitor and revalidate an established sterilization cycle.

Q21. Mention the recommended biological indicators, employed in autoclaving or steam sterilization.

Ans. Spores of *Bacillus stearothemophilus* or Clostridium *sporogenes*. The number of viable spores should be more than 10^5 per carrier.

Q22. Mention the recommended biological indicator employed in dry heat sterilization.

Ans. Spores of bacillus *subtilis*. The number of viable spores should be more than 10^5 per carrier.

4

Evaluation of Surgical Dressings

Exercise 18

OBJECT

Evaluation of given sample of absorbent cotton for acidity or alkalinity, identification and surface active substances as per IP (1996) norms.

Chemicals

Iodinated zinc chloride solution, zinc chloride solution, dilute phenolphthalein solution, methyl orange solution, sulphuric acid.

Principle

Absorbent cotton occurs as white, soft, well carded fibres, containing not more than traces of leaf residue, seed coat and other impurities. It is odourless, cleaned, purified and bleached. It does not contain any compensatory colouring matter.

All statements with monographs given under the heading "standard" constitute standards. The absorbents cotton is not of pharmacopoeial quality unless it complies with all of the requirements stated.

Procedure

Experiments	*Observation*	*Inference*
1. **Identification** Take a clean slide, place few cotton fibres on slide, put few drops of iodinated zinc chloride solution on fibres and examined under microscope.	Violet colour fibres are seen.	Cotton fibres are present.

(Contd.)

Experiments		*Observation*	*Inference*
2.	**Acidity or alkalinity** To 15 g add 150 ml of water, Macerate for 2 hours in a closed vessel, decant the liquid, carefully squeezing out the residual liquid with a glass rod. Mix and filter (Solution-A), To 25 ml of filterate add 0.1 ml of dilute phenolphthalein solution, to another 25 ml add 0.05 ml of methyl orange solution.	Neither solutions show a pink colour.	passes the test.
3.	**Surface active substances** Take graduated glass stoppered cylinder (25 ml), which is previously rinsed with sulphuric acid and then with water, add 10 ml of solution-A (reserved in the test for acidity or alkalinity), shake vigorously 30 times in 10 seconds, allow to stand for 1 minute and shake again 30 times. After 5 minutes the height of the froth is measured. (External diameter of the above graduated cylinder should be of 18 to 22 mm).	The height of the froth does not exceed 2 mm above the surface of the liquid.	passes the test.

Result

Identification	–	Passes/does not pass
Acidity or alkalinity	–	Passes/does not pass
Surface active substances	–	Passes/does not pass

Reagent

Iodinated zinc chloride solution

Dissolve 20 g of zinc chloride and 6.5 g of potassium iodide in 10.5 ml of water. Add 0.5 g of iodine and shake for 15 minutes. Filter if necessary.

Exercise 19

OBJECT

Evaluation of given sample of absorbent cotton for neps, fluorescence and colouring matter as per IP (1996) norms.

Chemicals

Ethanol 95%, hydrochloric acid, cupric sulphate, colorimetric solution (CSS) acetic acid, potassium iodide, sodium thiosulphate, starch solution.

Principle

Absorbent cotton occurs as white, soft, well carded fibres, containing not more than traces of leaf residue, seed coat and other impurities. It is odourless, cleaned, purified and bleached. It does not contain any compensatory colouring matter.

All statements with monographs given under the heading "standard" constitute standards. The absorbents cotton is not of pharmacopoeial quality unless it complies with all of the requirements stated.

Procedure

1. **Neps** Take 0.5 g of absorbent cotton and spread uniformly between two glass plates in thin layer for an area of 450 sq cm and view by the necked eye under transmitted light. Count the number of neps for the above whole area. Repeat the test three times and calculate the average number of neps.	1. The average number of neps does not exceed 250 2. If the average number of neps exceed 250	Passes the test Does not pass
2. **Fluorescence** Examine a layer about 5 mm in thickness under ultraviolet light (365 nm)	It shows only a slight brownish violet fluorescence and a few yellow particles. Not more than few isolated fibres show an intense blue fluorescence.	Passes the test
3. **Colouring matter** Slowly extract 10 g in a narrow percolator with ethanol (95%) until 50 ml of extract is obtained. The extract is not more intensely coloured than a solution prepared in the following manner. Standard solution. To 3 ml of CSS add 7 ml of a solution of hydrochloric acid containing 1% W/V of HCl and dilute 0.5 ml of the resulting solution to 10 ml with the same solution of HCl.	(i) The extract solution is not more intense than that of standard solution (ii) The extract solution is intense than that of standard solution.	Passes the test Does not pass

Result

Neps	–	Passes/ does not pass
Fluorescence	-	Passes/ does not pass
Colouring matter	–	Passes/ does not pass

Reagents

Cupric sulphate colorimetric solution (CSS)

Dissolve about 65 g of cupric sulphate in enough of a mixture of 25 ml of hydrochloric acid and 975 ml of water to produce 1000 ml. Pipette 10 ml of this solution in to a 250 ml iodine flask, add 40 ml of water, 4 ml of acetic acid, 3 g of potassium iodide and 5 ml of hydrochloric acid. Titrate the liberated iodine with 0.1M sodium thiosulphate solution using 0.5 ml of starch solution, added towards the pale brown end point, as indicator. Perform a blank determination and make necessary correction.

Each ml of 0.1M sodium thiosulphate is equivalent to 0.02497 g of $CuSO_4\,5H_2O$. Adjust the final volume of the solution by addition of enough of the mixture of hydrochloric acid and water so that each ml contains 0.0624 g of $CuSO_4\,5H_2O$.

Acetic acid

Contains approximately 33% W/W of acetic acid. Dilute 315 ml glacial acetic acid to 1000 ml with water.

Starch solution: Triturate 1 g of soluble starch with 5 ml of water and add, stirring continuously, to 100 ml of boiling water containing 10 mg of mercuric iodide.

Sodium thiosulphate (0.1M)

Dissolve 25 g of sodium thiosulphate and 0.2 g of sodium carbonate in carbon dioxide free water and dilute to 1000 ml with the same solvent. Standardize the solution.

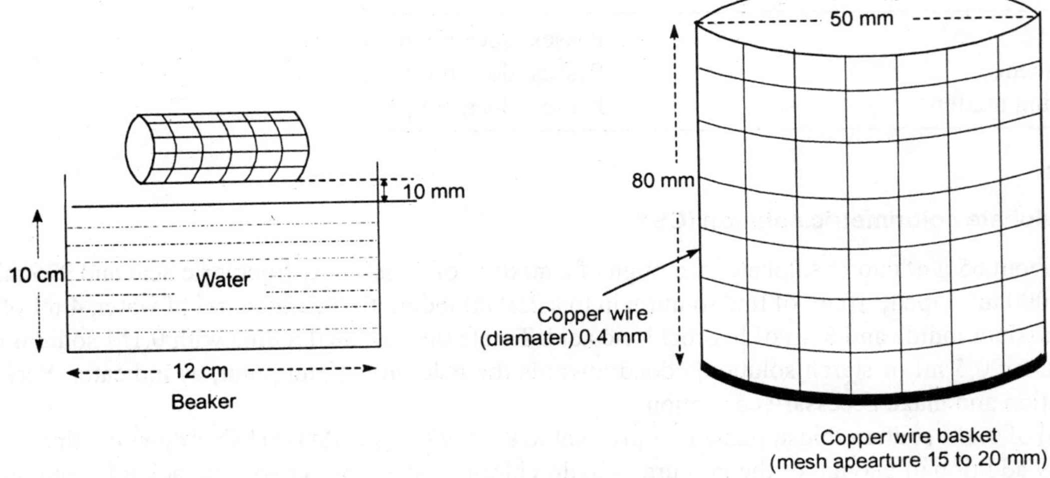
10 mm
10 cm
Water
12 cm
Beaker
50 mm
80 mm
Copper wire
(diamater) 0.4 mm
Copper wire basket
(mesh apearture 15 to 20 mm)

Fig. 4

Exercise 20

OBJECT

Evaluation of given sample of absorbent cotton for absorbency (sinking time and water holding capacity) as per IP (1996) norms.

Apparatus

Beaker, copper wire, basket, stop watch and absorbent cotton.

Principle

Absorbent cotton should be stored in cool place otherwise improper storage condition may result in loss of its absorbent power due to intramolecular rearrangement. Bacterial attack makes it brittle and dusty. Indian pharmacopoeia mentions two parameters, i.e. sinking time and water holding capacity, under the test absorbency.

Sinking time should be not more than 10 seconds while water holding capacity should not less than 23 g per g of sample.

Procedure

Experiments	*Observation*	*Inference*
Sinking time Weigh the basket accurately. Take five sample of absorbent cotton being examined each of approximately 1 g from different places, pack loosely in the basket and weigh the packed basket. Hold the basket with its long axis in the horizontal position and drop its from a height of about 10 mm in to water at 25° C contained in a beaker (Fig. 4). Measure with stop watch the time taken by the basket to sink below the surface of water. Repeat the procedure on two further samples and calculate the average value of the three readings.	(i) Sinking time should be not more than 10 seconds. (ii) If sinking time is more than 10 seconds.	Passes the test Does not pass
Water Holding capacity Remove the basket from the water of above experiment, allow it to drain for 30 seconds with its long axis in the horizontal position, transfer it to a tared (already weighed)	(i) Water holding capacity should not less than 23 gram per gram of sample. (ii) If it is more than 23 g per gram of sample.	Passes the test Does not pass

(Contd.)

Experiments	*Observation*	*Inference*
beaker and weigh. calculate the weigh of water retained by the sample. Repeat the procedure on two further samples and calculate the average value.		

Result

Sinking time	–	Passes/does not pass
Water holding capacity	–	Passes/does not pass

Calculation

1. Weight of basket	–	a gram
2. Weight of basket + dry cotton	–	b gram
3. Weight of basket + wet cotton	–	c gram
4. Weight of water retained	–	(c-b) gram
5. Weight of cotton	–	b-a gram
6. Weight of water retained per gram of cotton sample	–	(c-b) /(b-a)

Note

Take further two reading in similar manner and calculate the average of the three readings.

Exercise 21

OBJECT

Evaluation of given sample of absorbent cotton for ether soluble substances and water soluble substances as per IP 1996 norms.

Apparatus

Soxhlet apparatus, beaker, glass rod.

Chemical

Ether.

Principle

Since raw cotton contains waxy matter and other impurities, so it is subject to process of combing, boiling with dilute caustic soda solution, washing and drying, etc.

The Indian pharmacopoeia states that the official absorbent cotton should contained not more than traces of leaf residue, seed coat and other impurities. It does not contain any compensatory colouring matter. So Indian pharmacopoeia mentions the limit for ether soluble and water soluble substances. For each extract, it should not be more than 0.5%.

Procedure

Ether soluble substances

Extract 5 g with ether in a soxhlet apparatus for four hours in such a way that the rate is at least four extracts per hour. Evaporate the ether and dry the residue to constant weight at 105° C.

Water soluble substances

Boil 5 g with 500 ml of water for 30 minutes, stirring frequently and replacing the water loss by evaporation. Decant the liquid in to a beaker, squeeze the residual liquid from the material carefully with a glass rod, mix the liquids and filter the extract whilst hot. Evaporate 400 ml of filterate and dry the residue to constant weight at 105° C.

Result

Ether soluble substances	–	Passes /does not pass
Water soluble substances	–	Passes/does not pass

Exercise 22

OBJECT

Evaluation of given sample of absorbent cotton for loss on drying as per IP 1996 norms.

Apparatus

Absorbent cotton, weighing bottle, oven.

Principle

Loss in drying is the loss in weight in percentage W/W is resulting from water and volatile matter of any kind that can be driven off under specific conditions. The Indian pharmacopoeia has specified that loss on drying should not be more than 8% W/W.

% Loss on drying

$$= \frac{\text{weight loss (weight of moisture present in given sample)}}{\text{weight of sample (absorbent cotton)}} \times 100$$

Procedure

Weigh glass stoppered shallow weighing bottle that has been dried in oven at 105° C. Take 5 g of sample being examined in the bottle, cover it and accurately way the bottle and content. The distribution of sample should be evenly. Place the loaded bottle in the oven at 105° C, remove the stopper and leave it also in the chamber. Dry the sample to constant weight at 105° C. After drying is completed, open the drying chamber, close the bottle and allow it to cool to room temperature in a oven. Weigh the bottle and sample. Calculate the % loss on drying in W/W.

Result

Viva Voce

Q1. Define surgical dressings.

Ans. All the materials which are used for the dressing of wounds and favour their healing is called surgical dressings.

Q2. Classify surgical dressings.

Ans. They are classified as follow

(i) *Fibres:* Absorbent cotton, silk, etc.

(ii) *Fabric:* Absorbent lint, absorbent ribbon gauze, etc.

(iii) *Bandages:* Crepe bandage, elastic bandage, etc.

(iv) *Rubber and oil in impregnated material:* Belladonna self adhesive plaster.

Q3. Enlist the types of surgical dressings as recognized by B.P.

Ans. (i) *Fibres and related materials:* viscose.

(ii) *Carded products:* absorbent cotton

(iii) Non-extensible, nonadhesive woven products: absorbent muslin

(iv) Non-extensible adhesive woven products: absorbent-belladonna adhesive plaster.

(v) Extensible nonadhesive products: cotton bandage.

(vi) Extensible adhesive woven products: elastic adhesive bandage.

(vii) Non-woven products: impermeable plastic surgical adhesive tape.

Q4. What is neps?

Ans. Neps are entangled masses of fibres visible to naked eye. Excess moisture content gives rise to more number of neps. It is official test.

Q5. What is naps?

Ans. This refers to loose fibres which makes the cotton lint weakened.

Q6. What is yarn?

Ans. The thread is prepared by spinning of fibres ıs termed as yarn.

Q7. What is slubs?

Ans. Thick soft parts of a yarn is called slubs.

Q8. What is warp and weft?

Ans. The longitudinal threads of cotton fabric is called warp while horizontal threads are crossed at right angle to warp is called weft.

Q9. What is lint?

Ans. It is a cloth of plain weave in which the warp threads are cotton and weft may contain cotton or a mixture of cotton and regenerated fibres, used as absorbent and protective dressing.

Q10. Write the biological source of absorbent cotton.

Ans. It consists of epidermal hairs of the seeds of *Gossypium herbaceum* and other species belong to Malvaceae family.

Q11. Write functions of surgical dressings.

Ans. (i) It favours healing of wounds.

(ii) It provides physical protection to wounds.

(iii) It also provides mechanical support to surrounding tissues.

Q12. Write properties of surgical dressings.

Ans. (i) It should be free from loose threads ends and fibres.

(ii) It should not adhere to the wound surface.

(iii) It should be durable and easy to handle.
(iv) Sterilization should be easy.

Q13. What is primary wound dressings?

Ans. They are applied over the surface of wound to absorb pus, mucus and blood. Example–viscose gauze.

Q14. Define bandage.

Ans. It is a material which holds dressings in required place to provide pressure or support and prevents bleeding. It may be elastic or non-elastic in nature. Examples–common gauze roller bandage, muslin bandage, crepe bandage, etc.

Q15. What is surgical gauze?

Ans. It is material to provide an absorbent property of sufficient tensile strength for surgical dressings. It is classified according to its mesh or number of threads per 10 cm.

Q16. Enlist standards for surgical gauze which is official in BP but not in IP.

Ans. (i) Threads per 10 cm.
(ii) Weight per unit area.
(iii) Yarn number.
(iv) Minimum breaking load.

Q17. What are protectives?

Ans. They are employed to cover wet dressings to prevent the loss of moisture or heat from wounds. Example–plastic sheet, waxed or plastic coated paper.

Q18. What is suture and ligature?

Ans. Surgical suture is a thread used for sewing or stitching together tissues, muscles and tendons with the help of a needle.

Ligature is thread used to tie a blood vessels to stop bleeding without the use of a needle.

Q19. Write the limit of absorbent cotton for sinking time and water holding capacity as IP norms.

Ans. Sinking time–It should not be more than 10 seconds.

Water holding capacity–It should not be less than 23 g per g of a sample being examined.

Q20. Write importance of fluorescence test for absorbent cotton.

Ans. IP recommends that the absorbent cotton does not contain any compensatory colouring matter. So to know the extent of presence of colouring matter fluorescence test is carried out.

5

Handling and Use of Data Processing Equipments

Various types of data processing equipment are available nowadays and calculator is the simplest form of data processing equipment, but it can only perform basic mathematical operations. Knowledge obtained from analysis of available data is a need of modern days for each profession. In the modern time to collect latest, up to date and arranged information by processing of available data, computer is the only powerful medium. Computer is an electronic device which process raw data to give meaningful information. Computers are machines, which can do a variety of jobs very quickly; these are fast working and can do calculations and analyses of a very large data in fraction of seconds for which a human being may take many days. Computers can store the information as well.

This is the age of computer. Computers are more popular these days because of its capabilities in terms of speed, accuracy and versatility. Nowadays in medical profession and hospitals, computers are used by doctors and pharmacist to gain up-to-date knowledge about details of patient, disease, inventory control and storage details of medicines and equipment, preparation of reports of pathological tests, etc. Information obtained by data analysis is:

- Helpful for updating of knowledge
- Helpful in decision making
- Helpful for future planning

Anatomy of a computer system

Computer system can be divided in the following two parts

A. Hardware B. Software

Hardware

These include the mechanical, electrical and electronic part of the system. All physical parts of the computer system are collectively known as Hardware, e.g. monitor, mouse, keyboard, printers, microprocessors and motherboard, etc.

Software

Collection of different programmes that instruct a computer how to process the data and generate required information is called software. These are also helpful for contact between human (user) and computer. The methods and programmes used to create link between human and computer is called computer language.

(A) HARDWARE

Functional components of computer systems

Hardware of a computer system can be classified as follows:

(a) Central processing Unit (CPU).
(b) Peripherals.

(a) Central processing unit (CPU)

Processor or the brain part of the computer system, it is composed of following units:

(i) Control unit

This unit controls all part of the computer system, it deals with the input as per the instructions using the memory. After processing it sends results back to memory and from memory to output devices.

(ii) Memory unit

When any data/information fed into the computer it is first sends to the memory and stored there.

(iii) Arithmetical and logical unit

In this unit, problems are duly processed and results are produced in required manner.

(b) Peripherals

It includes various devices attached to the CPU to feed data in CPU. These can be divided as:

(i) Input Devices (ii) Output Devices (iii) Storage Devices

(i) Input devices

With the help of input devices user feed data into the computer, e.g. key board, mouse, light pen, scanner, camera, Recorder, etc.

(ii) Output devices

These devices are used to output results to the user, e.g. monitor (Colourea or Black and White), Printers (Coloured inkjet, Dot matrix, laser), Speakers, etc.

(iii) Storage devices

These devices are used to store the data, programme and software permanently. Main storage devices are hard disk, Floppy, Compact disk (CD), etc.

Input (keyboard, mouse, etc.)→	Memory Unit (MU) Control Unit (CU) Arithmetic and logical Unit (ALU) CPU	→ Output unit (Printers, Monitors, etc.)

Like human brain, computer also stores information (data and Programmes) in memory. There are two types of memory in computer systems:-

(a) Internal or Primary memory (b) External or Secondary Memory

Internal and primary memory

working of computer depends upon the combination of two points, called puls, i.e. 1 and 0 . Different combinations of these puls produce different type of code like 0101, 0111, 1001010, etc. It is called binary digit system. One digit is called 1 bit. In storage device every key possess a different code of 8 bit. The puls rate is called the speed of computer and it is the basic unit of storage capacity of a computer, as given below –

8 bit	=	1 byte
1024 bytes	=	1 kilo byte (kB)
1024 kilo bytes	=	1 Mega byte (MB)
1024 Mega bytes	=	1 Gega byte (GB), etc.

The internal memory of computer is of two types:

(a) Random Access Memory (RAM).
(b) Read Only Memory. (ROM).

(a) RAM

It is like a black board in a class room on which information can be written, erased and rewrite, while rewriting data, previous data is erased, after switching off the computer RAM erased. Data can be written only on to the RAM.

(b) ROM

There are certain essential functions that the computer must perform when it is switched on, like establishing connection within various components of the computer and its peripherals. It is permanent memory for fixed instructions. It does not permit the user to write on it.

2. External memory

These are secondary devices meant for storing the programmes and data that has to be used at a later stage. Following are the examples of secondary/external storage devices.

1. Floppy disk
2. Hard disk
3. Compact disk
4. Magnetic tape, etc.

(B) SOFTWARE

Software of a computer system can be classified as follows

(a) System software
(b) Application software
(c) Utility software
(d) General purpose software

System Software

This type of software allows contact of computer with different peripheral devices, e.g. Monitors, Printers, etc. These are the base of application software. These are also helpful in preparation of other software also, e.g. Operation system like Windows(98 and XP, etc.), Disk Operating system (DOS), Linex and Interpreter, etc.

Application Software

Such software are designed for doing particular job on computer, e.g. Tally for accounting purpose, software for preparing salaries, etc.

Utility Software

Such software are programmed for maintenance of computer, e.g. Disk recovery software, Antivirus software, etc.

General purpose Software

These software are prepared for general use, e.g. MS Office containing MS Word, MS Excel, etc.

Following are the computer related terms

Abacus : The earliest calculating machine was a manual device called abacus.
ALU : The problems are duly processed and the decisions are taken.
Calculator : A device that can perform basic mathematical operations.
Control Unit : This unit controls all the parts of the computer.
CPU : The heart of computer is called CPU.
Cursor : The screen is always displaying white flashing line that keeps on blinking till the computer system is switched off, called cursor.
Data : Unarranged and unorganized factor and figure, which we feed to the computers.
Hardware : A name given to the physical parts of a computer collectively'.
Information : The final result obtains by the computer after processing the data with the help of a programme.
Memory : The area inside the computer where the information is stored.
Peripheral : The devices are attached to the CPU at its periphery called Peripheral.
Program : A set of instructions loaded into memory of the computer or the set of instructions given to the computer for analysis or rearrangement of data to produce meaningful information is called programme.
Software : It is a collection of Programs that instruct a computer how to process the data and generate required information.

Exercise 23

OBJECT

Preparation of patient's profile for single patient in MS Word.

1. Name of the Patient	— Navin Singh.
2. Age of Patient	— 21 years.
3. Sex	— Male.
4. Chief complaint	— Cough with sputum, mild pain in abdomen and poor evacuation.
5. History of present illness (HOPI)	— Cough with sputum for last 3 days. Mild intermittent pain in abdomen, after taking meals or early in the morning for last 4 days.
6. History of past illness	— Not significant.
7. Occupational History	— Student.
8. Treatment History	— Not significant.
9. Physical Examination	— Mild epigastric pain. Pain in throat.
10. Diagnosis	— Throat infection and hyperacidity.
11. Treatment	— Ocid 20, Ciza MPS, Geri OZ, Levo-citrazine.
12. Other	— Patient should avoid dust, smoke and sore and cold things in meals.

Steps for opening MS Word

- Start the computer
- Click the start button in the bottom-left corner of window desktop (see Fig. 1).
- Click the programs choice on the resulting menu.
- Click the Microsoft Word choice in the menu (see Fig. 2).
- This will run Word and start a new document using default settings (see Fig. 3).
- You can set type and size of font. (see Fig. 4 and 5).
- Start typing the given exercise.

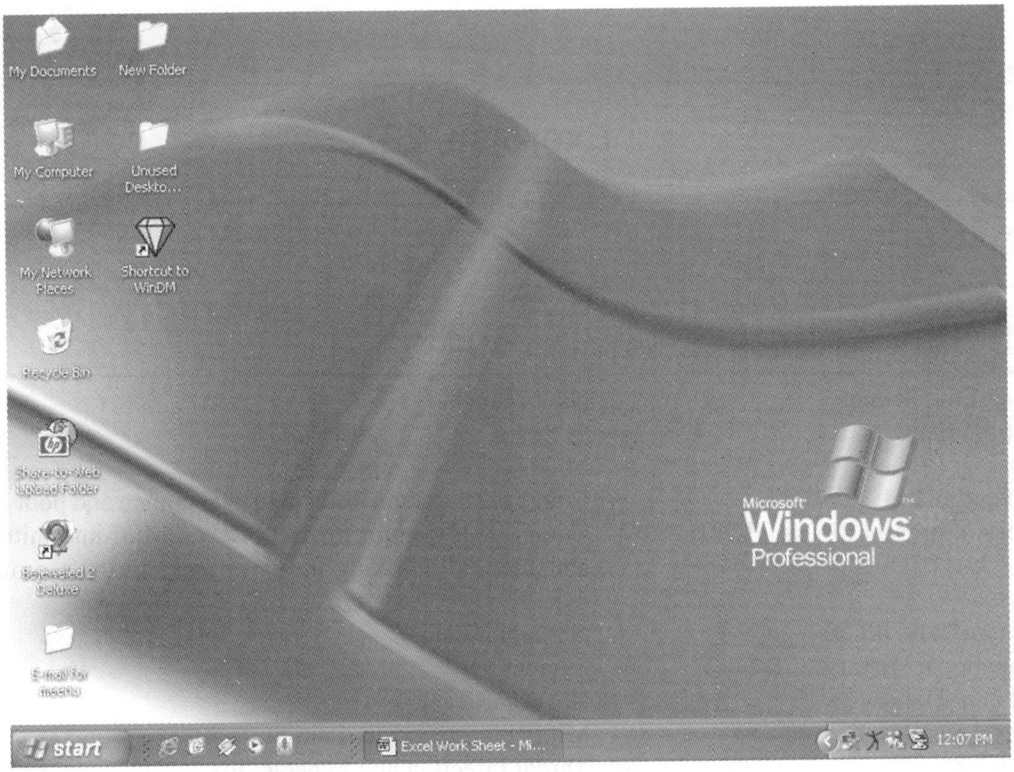
My Documents
New Folder
My Computer
Unused Deskto...
My Network Places
Shortcut to WinDM
Recycle Bin
Share-to-Web Upload Folder
Bejeweled 2 Deluxe
E-mail for meenu
Microsoft Windows Professional
start
Excel Work Sheet - Mi...
12:07 PM

Fig. 1

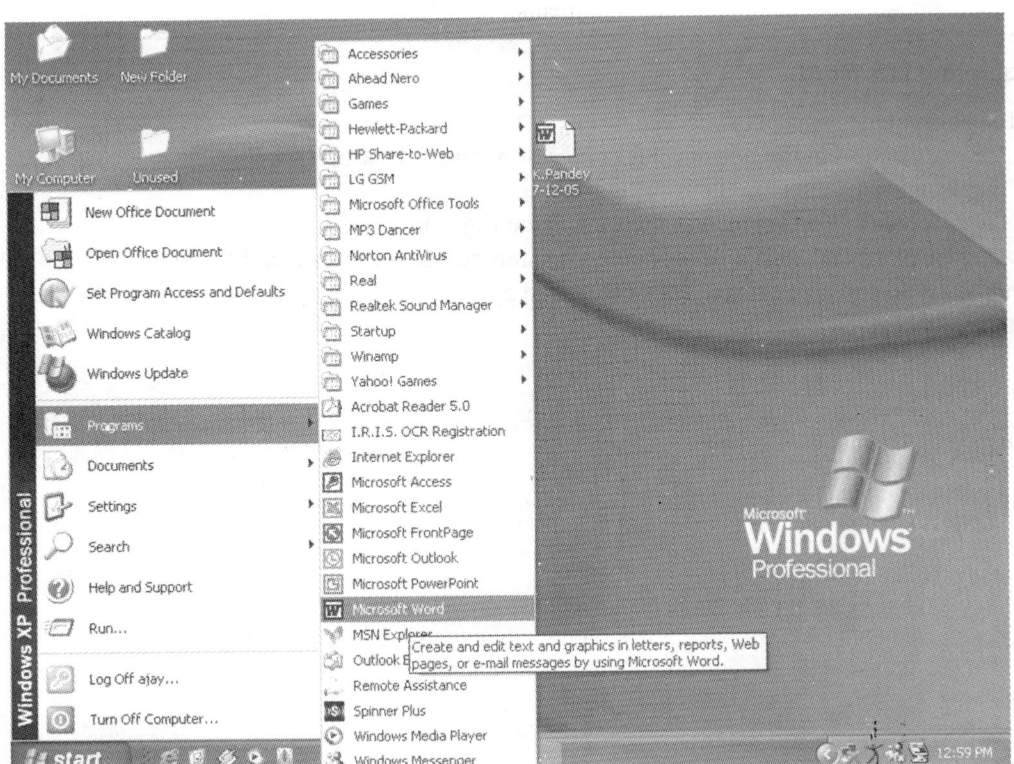
My Documents
New Folder
My Computer
Unused
K.Pandey 7-12-05
New Office Document
Open Office Document
Set Program Access and Defaults
Windows Catalog
Windows Update
Programs
Documents
Settings
Search
Help and Support
Run...
Log Off ajay...
Turn Off Computer...
Windows XP Professional
Accessories
Ahead Nero
Games
Hewlett-Packard
HP Share-to-Web
LG GSM
Microsoft Office Tools
MP3 Dancer
Norton AntiVirus
Real
Realtek Sound Manager
Startup
Winamp
Yahoo! Games
Acrobat Reader 5.0
I.R.I.S. OCR Registration
Internet Explorer
Microsoft Access
Microsoft Excel
Microsoft FrontPage
Microsoft Outlook
Microsoft PowerPoint
Microsoft Word
MSN Explorer
Create and edit text and graphics in letters, reports, Web pages, or e-mail messages by using Microsoft Word.
Remote Assistance
Spinner Plus
Windows Media Player
Windows Messenger
Microsoft Windows Professional
start
12:59 PM

Fig. 2

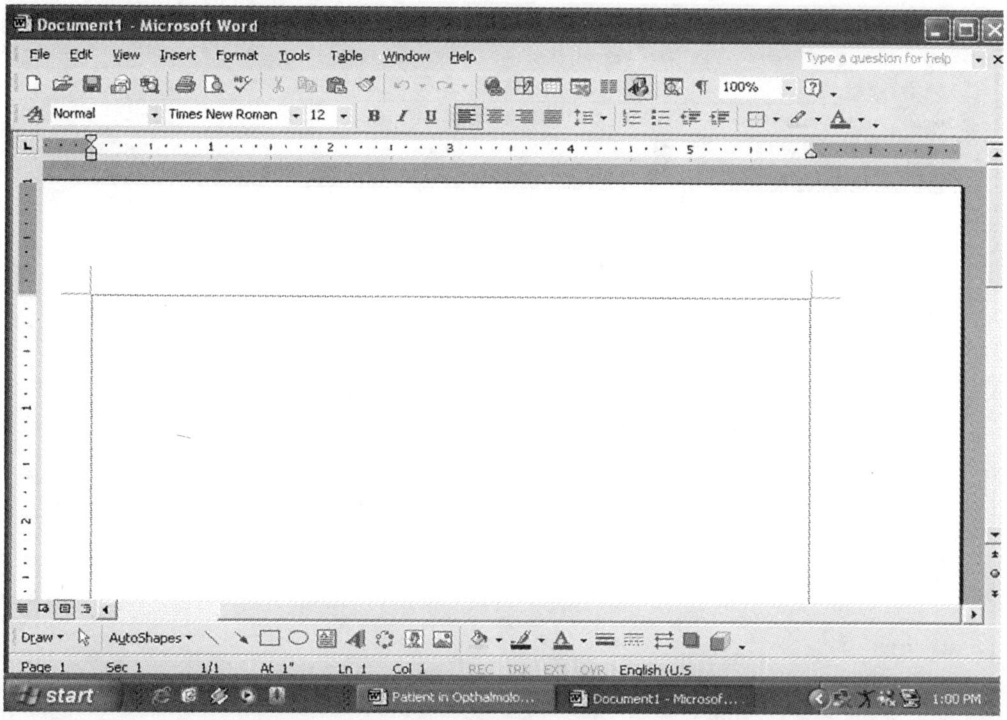
Document1 - Microsoft Word
File Edit View Insert Format Tools Table Window Help
Type a question for help
Normal
Times New Roman
12
100%
Draw
AutoShapes
Page 1 Sec 1 1/1 At 1" Ln 1 Col 1 REC TRK EXT OVR English (U.S
start
Patient in Opthalmolo...
Document1 - Microsof...
1:00 PM

Fig. 3

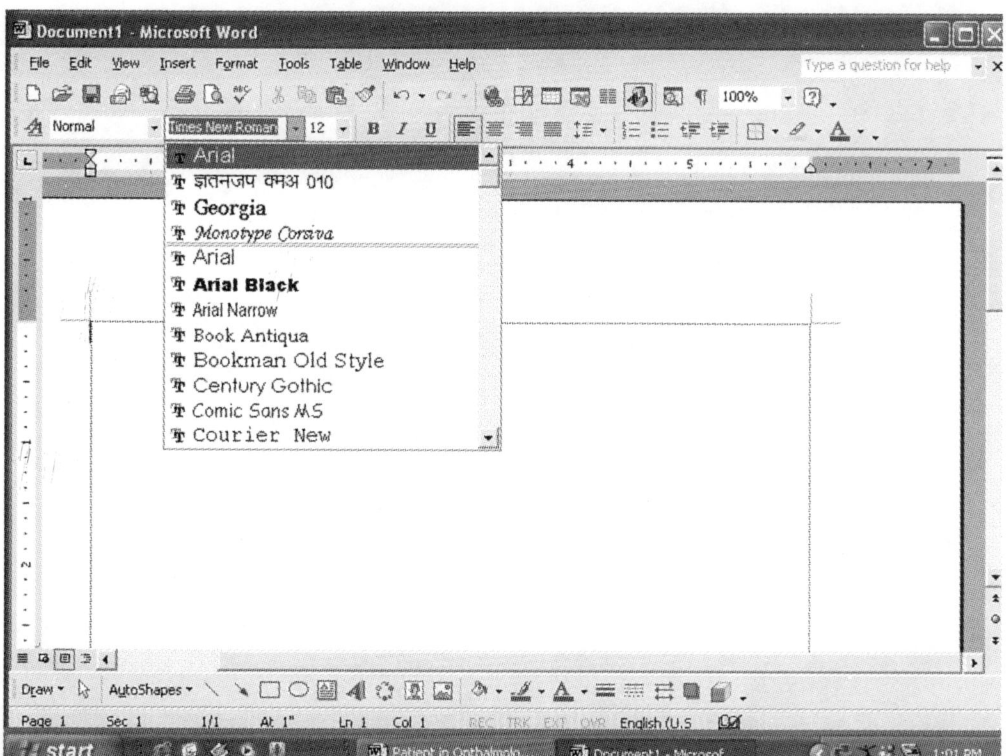
Document1 - Microsoft Word
File Edit View Insert Format Tools Table Window Help
Type a question for help
Normal
Times New Roman
12
100%
Arial
Georgia
Monotype Corsiva
Arial
Arial Black
Arial Narrow
Book Antiqua
Bookman Old Style
Century Gothic
Comic Sans MS
Courier New
Draw
AutoShapes
Page 1 Sec 1 1/1 At 1" Ln 1 Col 1 REC TRK EXT OVR English (U.S
start
Patient in Opthalmolo...
Document1 - Microsof...
1:01 PM

Fig. 4

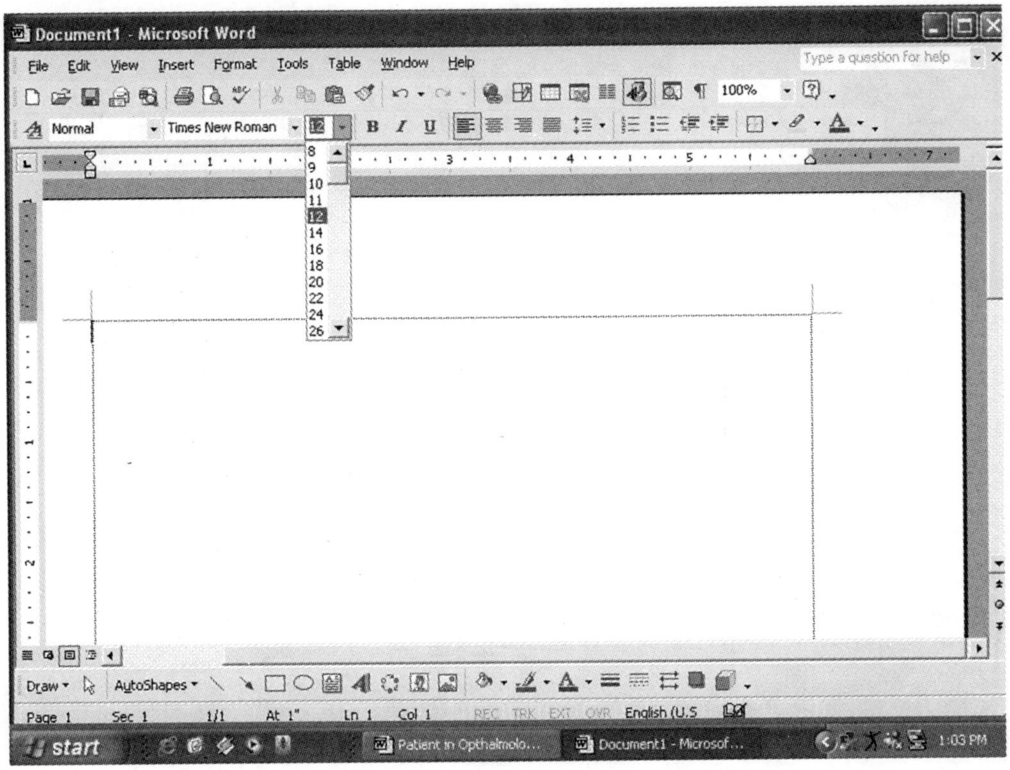
Document1 - Microsoft Word
File Edit View Insert Format Tools Table Window Help
Type a question for help
100%
Normal
Times New Roman
12
8
9
10
11
12
14
16
18
20
22
24
26
Draw
AutoShapes
Page 1 Sec 1 1/1 At 1" Ln 1 Col 1 REC TRK EXT OVR English (U.S
start
Patient in Opthalmolo...
Document1 - Microsof...
1:03 PM

Fig. 5

Exercise 24

OBJECT

Preparation of record for registration of patients in hospital using Microsoft Excel worksheet.
Registration of Patients in Hospital in Microsoft excel spread sheet

	NEW PATIENT						OLD PATIENT					
Date	*Reg.No.*	*S.No.*	*Name of patient*	*Age*	*Sex*	*Department*	*Reg.No*	*S.No.*	*Name of Patient*	*Age*	*Sex*	*Department*
9-Dec-05	8076	1	Mausim	22	M	Ophthalmology	7254	1	Shakuntala	40	F	Gyno & obst
9-Dec-05	8077	2	Rakesh	30	M	Medicin	7001	2	Santosh	30	M	Medicin
9-Dec-05	8078	3	Premlata	25	F	Ophthalmology	7005	3	Yameen	35	M	Ophthalmology
9-Dec-05	8079	4	Rajkumar	4	M	Ophthalmology	7014	4	Mamta	27	F	Gyno & obst
9-Dec-05	8080	5	Navin	30	F	Surgery	7019	5	D.K.Agarwal	35	M	Ophthalmology
9-Dec-05	8081	6	Satvir	22	M	Medicin	7036	6	Kapoori	65	F	Gyno & obst
9-Dec-05	8082	7	Shashi	40	F	Gyno & obst	7026	7	Prema Singh	40	M	Ophthalmology
9-Dec-05	8083	8	Jamila	30	F	Ophthalmology	7034	8	Omvati	40	F	Medicin
10-Dec-05	8084	9	Neel Kamal	30	M	Medicin	7467	9	Billo	40	F	Gyno & obst
10-Dec-05	8085	10	Shayjaha	30	F	Gyno & obst	7472	10	Ramvati	30	F	Gyno & obst
10-Dec-05	8086	11	Rameshwari	45	F	Medicin	7463	11	Ramesh Chand	30	M	Medicin
10-Dec-05	8087	12	Mahendrapal	30	M	Ophthalmology	7471	12	Naushad	25	F	Ophthalmology
10-Dec-05	8088	13	Ankit	4	M	Medicin	7477	13	Indra davi	30	F	Gyno & obst
10-Dec-05	8089	14	B.K.Agarwal	30	M	Medicin	7480	14	Madanpal Singh	40	M	Ophthalmology
10-Dec-05	8090	15	Munni Davi	30	F	Gyno & obst	7484	15	Rajni	22	F	Gyno & obst
10-Dec-05	8091	16	Partibha	40	F	Surgery	7493	16	Kailash	30	M	Medicin
10-Dec-05	8092	17	Dinesh	30	M	Ophthalmology	7497	17	Pinku	22	M	Medicin
10-Dec-05	8093	18	Kusum	35	F	Gyno & obst	7506	18	Suresh	30	M	Ophthalmology
10-Dec-05	8094	19	Anuj	6	M	Medicin	7503	19	Baby Rakhi	3	F	Pediatrics
10-Dec-05	8095	20	Sharif	30	M	Surgery	7523	20	Raghuvir Singh	40	M	Medicin
10-Dec-05	8096	21	Kusum	30	F	Gyno & obst	7528	21	Gajala	20	F	Surgery
10-Dec-05	8097	22	Savitri	30	F	Surgery	7531	22	Pardeep Jindal	40	M	Medicin
11-Dec-05	8098	23	Manoj Kumar	40	M	Medicin	7534	23	Shashi	35	F	Surgery
11-Dec-05	8099	24	Mamta	25	F	Ophthalmology	7539	24	Satyapal Singh	37	M	Ophthalmology
11-Dec-05	8100	25	Mahesh	30	M	Ophthalmology	7544	25	Satyavati	30	F	Surgery
11-Dec-05	8101	26	Shyam	30	M	Medicin	7552	26	Shashi gupta	30	F	Medicin
11-Dec-05	8102	27	Patram	60	M	Surgery						
11-Dec-05	8103	28	Mahesh Sharma	30	M	Medicin						
11-Dec-05	8104	29	Aditya	5	M	Surgery						
11-Dec-05	8105	30	Indrajit	30	M	Ophthalmology						
11-Dec-05	8106	31	Rahees	30	M	Surgery						
11-Dec-05	8107	32	Satyapal	40	M	Ophthalmology						

Steps for opening MS Excel work sheet

- Start the computer.
- Click the start button in the bottom-left corner of window desktop (see Fig. 1).
- Click the programs choice on the resulting menu.
- Click the Microsoft Excel choice in the menu (see Fig. 6).
- This will run Excel and start a new worksheet using default settings (see Fig. 7).
- You can set type and size of font.
- Start typing the given exercise (see Fig. 8 and 9).

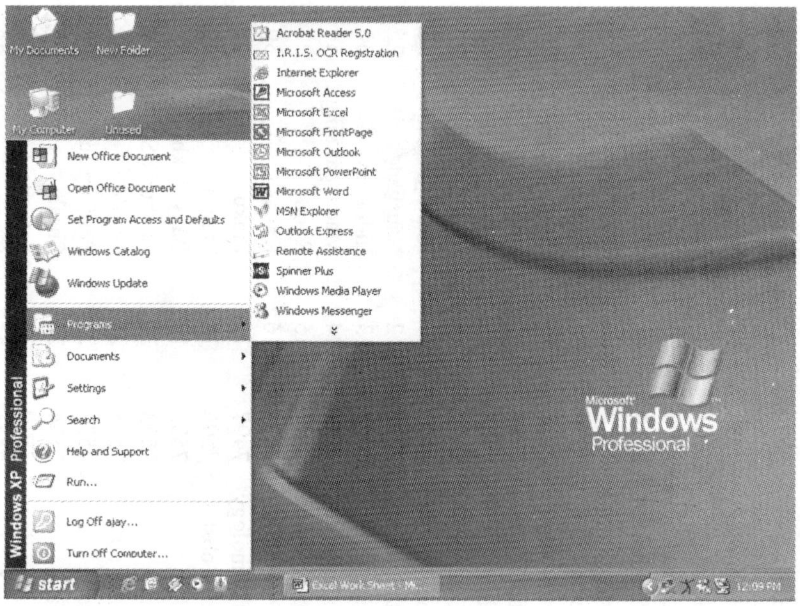

Fig. 6

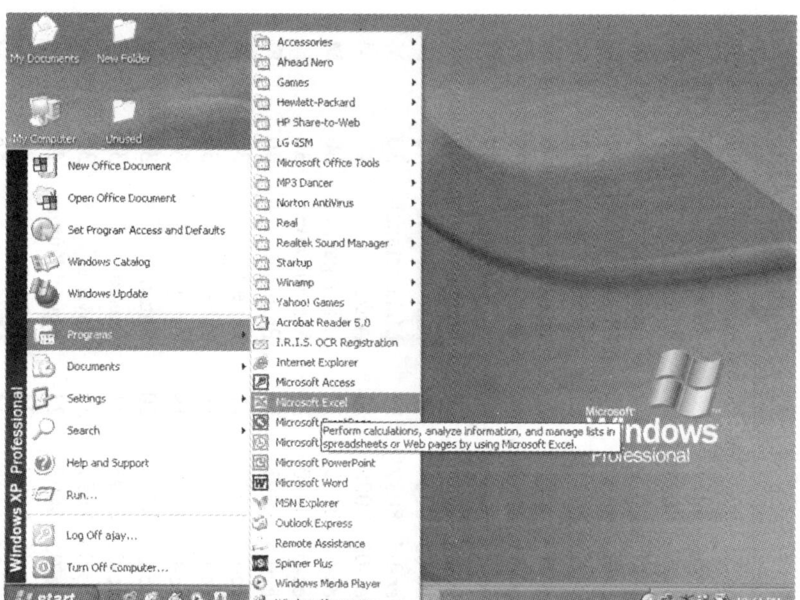

Fig. 7

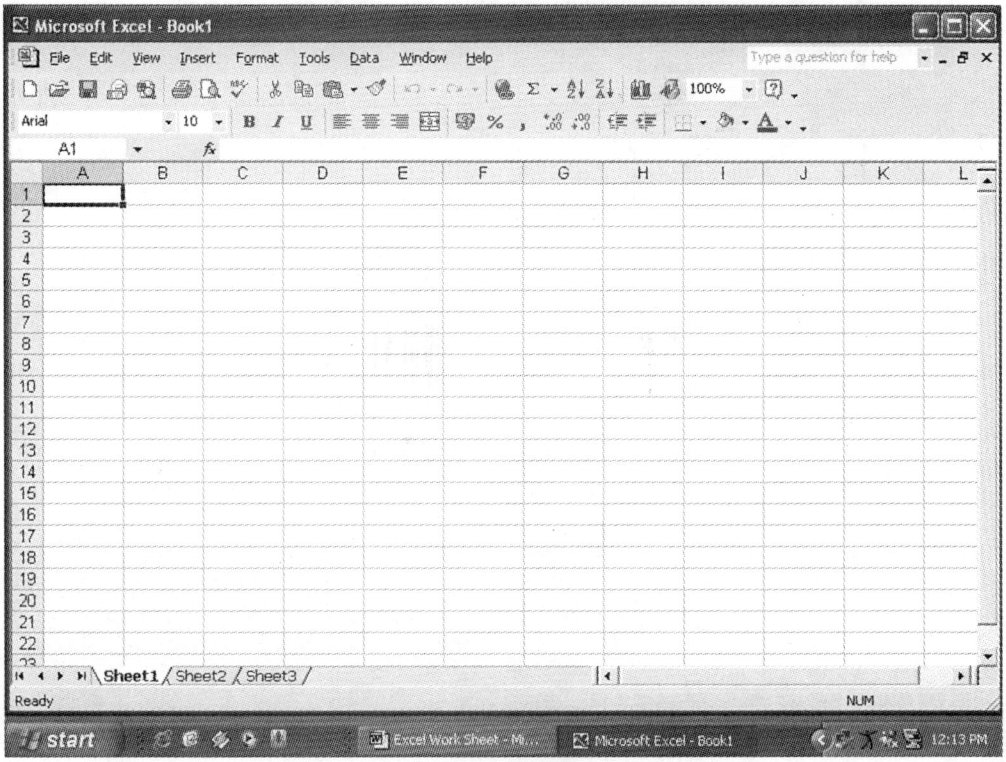
Microsoft Excel - Book1
File Edit View Insert Format Tools Data Window Help
Type a question for help
Arial
10
100%
A1
Sheet1 Sheet2 Sheet3
Ready
NUM
start
Excel Work Sheet - Mi...
Microsoft Excel - Book1
12:13 PM

Fig. 8

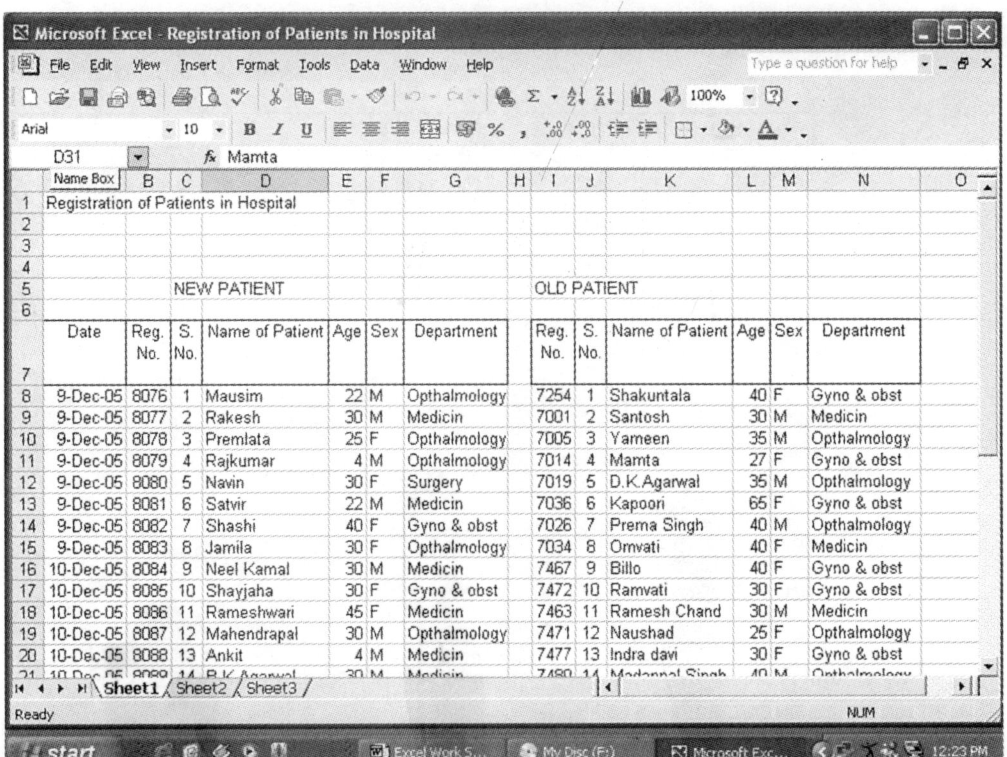
Microsoft Excel - Registration of Patients in Hospital
File Edit View Insert Format Tools Data Window Help
Type a question for help
Arial
10
100%
D31
Mamta
Name Box
Registration of Patients in Hospital
NEW PATIENT
OLD PATIENT
Date Reg. No. S. No. Name of Patient Age Sex Department
Reg. No. S. No. Name of Patient Age Sex Department
9-Dec-05 8076 1 Mausim 22 M Opthalmology 7254 1 Shakuntala 40 F Gyno & obst
9-Dec-05 8077 2 Rakesh 30 M Medicin 7001 2 Santosh 30 M Medicin
9-Dec-05 8078 3 Premlata 25 F Opthalmology 7005 3 Yameen 35 M Opthalmology
9-Dec-05 8079 4 Rajkumar 4 M Opthalmology 7014 4 Mamta 27 F Gyno & obst
9-Dec-05 8080 5 Navin 30 F Surgery 7019 5 D.K.Agarwal 35 M Opthalmology
9-Dec-05 8081 6 Satvir 22 M Medicin 7036 6 Kapoori 65 F Gyno & obst
9-Dec-05 8082 7 Shashi 40 F Gyno & obst 7026 7 Prema Singh 40 M Opthalmology
9-Dec-05 8083 8 Jamila 30 F Opthalmology 7034 8 Omvati 40 F Medicin
10-Dec-05 8084 9 Neel Kamal 30 M Medicin 7467 9 Billo 40 F Gyno & obst
10-Dec-05 8085 10 Shayjaha 30 F Gyno & obst 7472 10 Ramvati 30 F Gyno & obst
10-Dec-05 8086 11 Rameshwari 45 F Medicin 7463 11 Ramesh Chand 30 M Medicin
10-Dec-05 8087 12 Mahendrapal 30 M Opthalmology 7471 12 Naushad 25 F Opthalmology
10-Dec-05 8088 13 Ankit 4 M Medicin 7477 13 Indra davi 30 F Gyno & obst
Sheet1 Sheet2 Sheet3
Ready
NUM
start
Excel Work S...
My Disc (F:)
Microsoft Exc...
12:23 PM

Fig. 9

Exercise 25

OBJECT

Find out the name and number of new patients, above 30 years age, admitted in ophthalmology department of the hospital, using the data prepared in Exercise 24.

Steps for opening MS Excel work sheet

- Start the computer
- Open the worksheet prepared in exercise 24 (see Fig. 9).
- Click the data menu in title bar and click filter and than auto filter sub menu (see Fig. 10).
- Click on filter of Department column (see Fig. 11 and Fig. 12).
- Select Ophthalmology Department (see Fig. 13).
- Select the custom sub menu after opening filter of column of Age. A dialogue box will appear (see Fig. 14).
- In the dialogue box, select in Age box "is greater than" and "30" in the next box as shown in Fig. 15.
- Click OK Tab.
- See the result (Fig. 16).

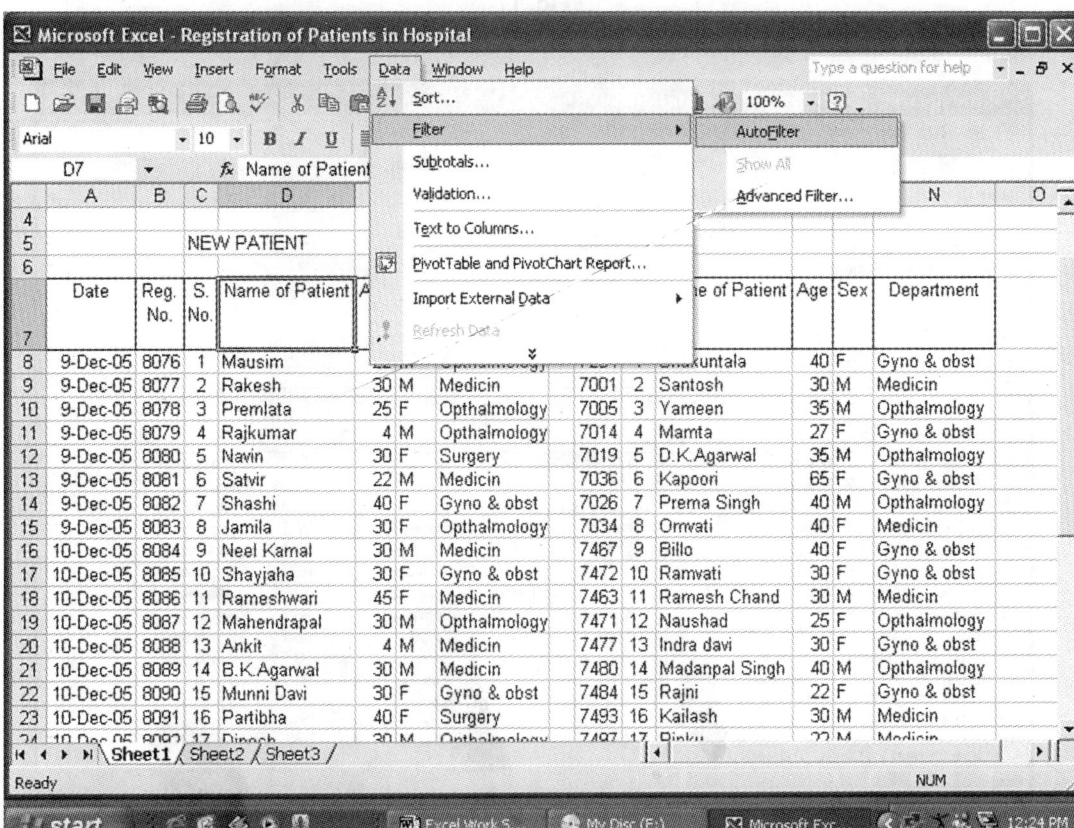

Fig. 10

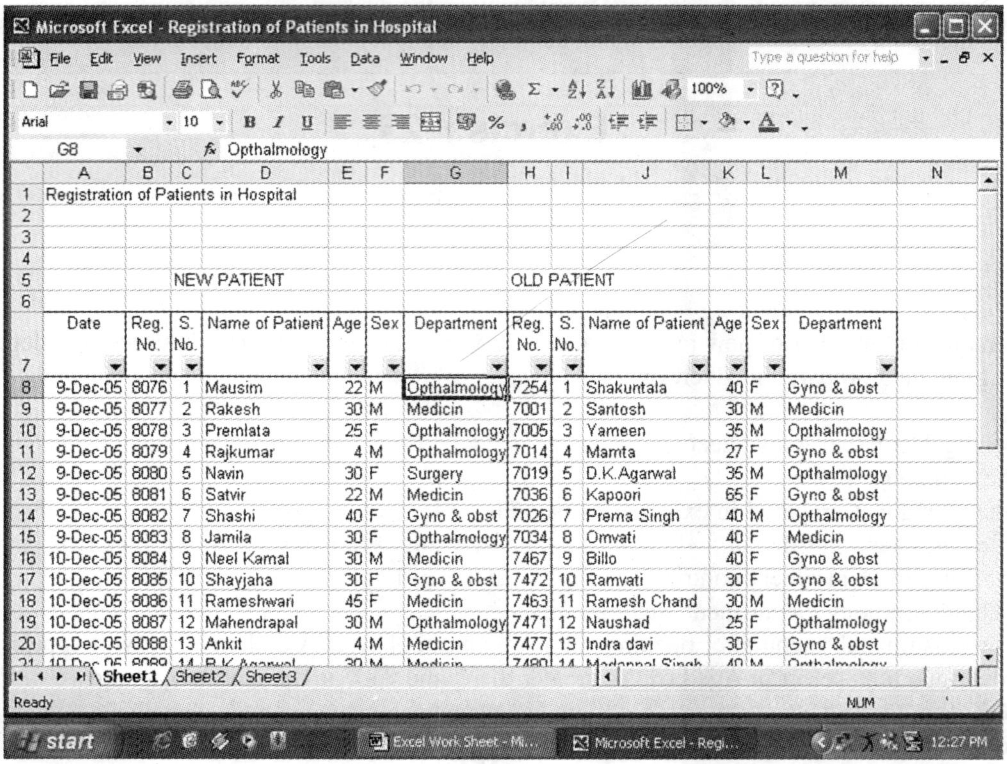

Date	Reg. No.	S. No.	Name of Patient	Age	Sex	Department	Reg. No.	S. No.	Name of Patient	Age	Sex	Department
9-Dec-05	8076	1	Mausim	22	M	Opthalmology	7254	1	Shakuntala	40	F	Gyno & obst
9-Dec-05	8077	2	Rakesh	30	M	Medicin	7001	2	Santosh	30	M	Medicin
9-Dec-05	8078	3	Premlata	25	F	Opthalmology	7005	3	Yameen	35	M	Opthalmology
9-Dec-05	8079	4	Rajkumar	4	M	Opthalmology	7014	4	Mamta	27	F	Gyno & obst
9-Dec-05	8080	5	Navin	30	F	Surgery	7019	5	D.K.Agarwal	35	M	Opthalmology
9-Dec-05	8081	6	Satvir	22	M	Medicin	7036	6	Kapoori	65	F	Gyno & obst
9-Dec-05	8082	7	Shashi	40	F	Gyno & obst	7026	7	Prema Singh	40	M	Opthalmology
9-Dec-05	8083	8	Jamila	30	F	Opthalmology	7034	8	Omvati	40	F	Medicin
10-Dec-05	8084	9	Neel Kamal	30	M	Medicin	7467	9	Billo	40	F	Gyno & obst
10-Dec-05	8085	10	Shayjaha	30	F	Gyno & obst	7472	10	Ramvati	30	F	Gyno & obst
10-Dec-05	8086	11	Rameshwari	45	F	Medicin	7463	11	Ramesh Chand	30	M	Medicin
10-Dec-05	8087	12	Mahendrapal	30	M	Opthalmology	7471	12	Naushad	25	F	Opthalmology
10-Dec-05	8088	13	Ankit	4	M	Medicin	7477	13	Indra davi	30	F	Gyno & obst

Fig. 11

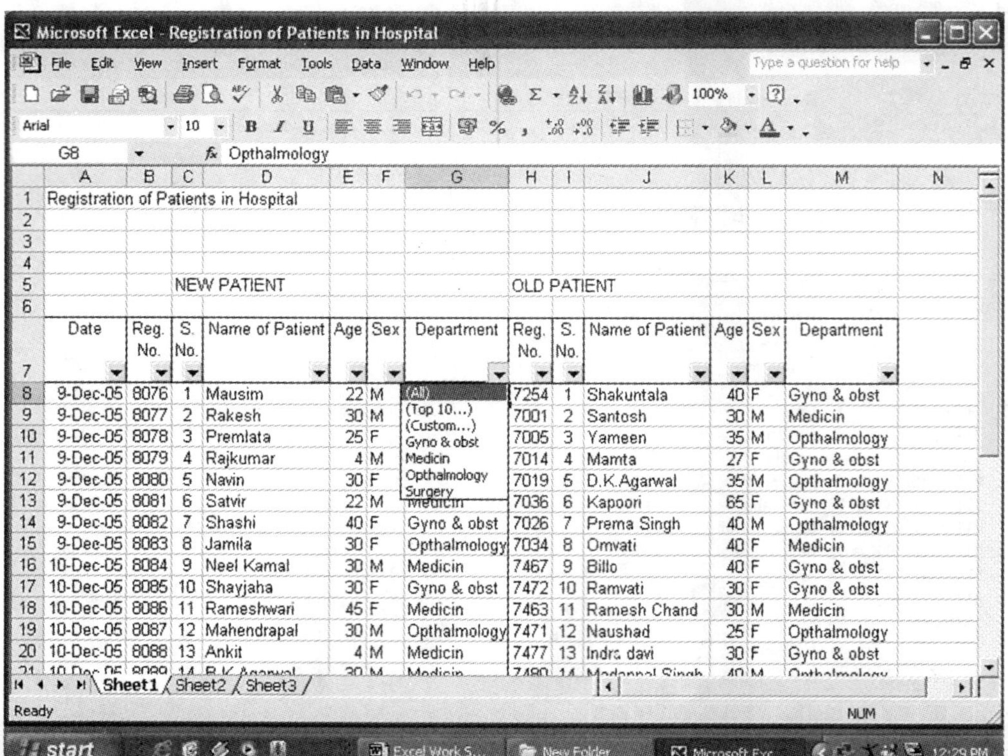

Date	Reg. No.	S. No.	Name of Patient	Age	Sex	Department	Reg. No.	S. No.	Name of Patient	Age	Sex	Department
9-Dec-05	8076	1	Mausim	22	M		7254	1	Shakuntala	40	F	Gyno & obst
9-Dec-05	8077	2	Rakesh	30	M		7001	2	Santosh	30	M	Medicin
9-Dec-05	8078	3	Premlata	25	F		7005	3	Yameen	35	M	Opthalmology
9-Dec-05	8079	4	Rajkumar	4	M		7014	4	Mamta	27	F	Gyno & obst
9-Dec-05	8080	5	Navin	30	F		7019	5	D.K.Agarwal	35	M	Opthalmology
9-Dec-05	8081	6	Satvir	22	M	Medicin	7036	6	Kapoori	65	F	Gyno & obst
9-Dec-05	8082	7	Shashi	40	F	Gyno & obst	7026	7	Prema Singh	40	M	Opthalmology
9-Dec-05	8083	8	Jamila	30	F	Opthalmology	7034	8	Omvati	40	F	Medicin
10-Dec-05	8084	9	Neel Kamal	30	M	Medicin	7467	9	Billo	40	F	Gyno & obst
10-Dec-05	8085	10	Shayjaha	30	F	Gyno & obst	7472	10	Ramvati	30	F	Gyno & obst
10-Dec-05	8086	11	Rameshwari	45	F	Medicin	7463	11	Ramesh Chand	30	M	Medicin
10-Dec-05	8087	12	Mahendrapal	30	M	Opthalmology	7471	12	Naushad	25	F	Opthalmology
10-Dec-05	8088	13	Ankit	4	M	Medicin	7477	13	Indra davi	30	F	Gyno & obst

Fig. 12

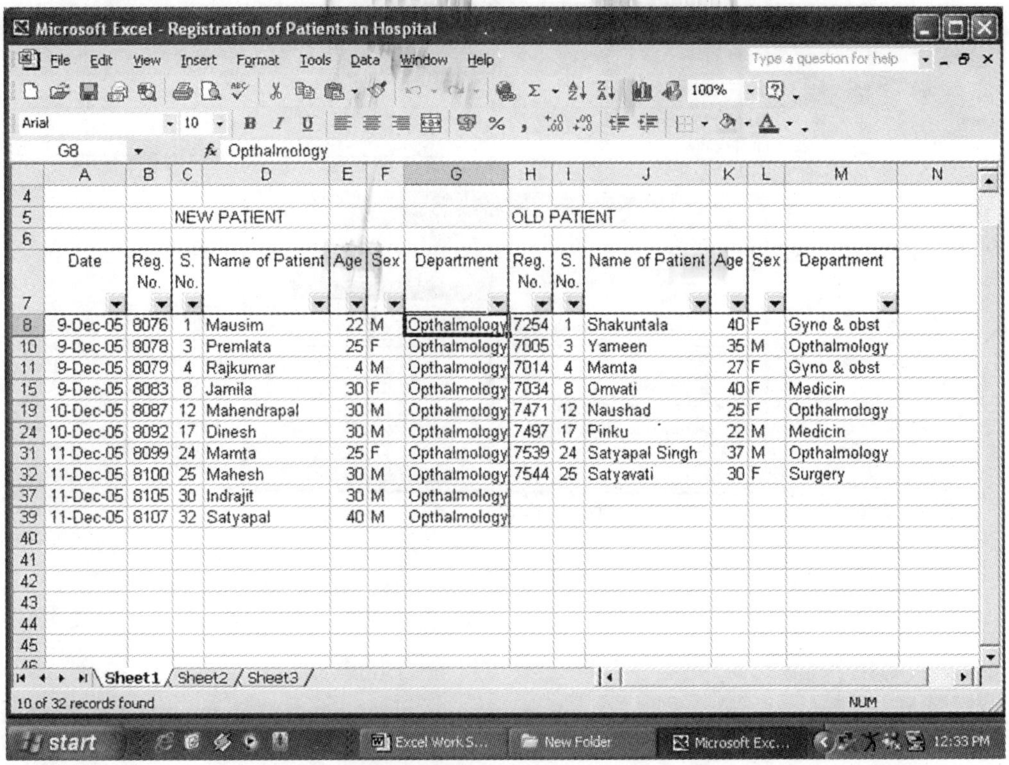
Microsoft Excel - Registration of Patients in Hospital
File Edit View Insert Format Tools Data Window Help
Type a question for help
Arial 10 100%
G8 Opthalmology
NEW PATIENT
OLD PATIENT
Date Reg. No. S. No. Name of Patient Age Sex Department Reg. No. S. No. Name of Patient Age Sex Department
9-Dec-05 8076 1 Mausim 22 M Opthalmology 7254 1 Shakuntala 40 F Gyno & obst
9-Dec-05 8078 3 Premlata 25 F Opthalmology 7005 3 Yameen 35 M Opthalmology
9-Dec-05 8079 4 Rajkumar 4 M Opthalmology 7014 4 Mamta 27 F Gyno & obst
9-Dec-05 8083 8 Jamila 30 F Opthalmology 7034 8 Omvati 40 F Medicin
10-Dec-05 8087 12 Mahendrapal 30 M Opthalmology 7471 12 Naushad 25 F Opthalmology
10-Dec-05 8092 17 Dinesh 30 M Opthalmology 7497 17 Pinku 22 M Medicin
11-Dec-05 8099 24 Mamta 25 F Opthalmology 7539 24 Satyapal Singh 37 M Opthalmology
11-Dec-05 8100 25 Mahesh 30 M Opthalmology 7544 25 Satyavati 30 F Surgery
11-Dec-05 8105 30 Indrajit 30 M Opthalmology
11-Dec-05 8107 32 Satyapal 40 M Opthalmology
Sheet1 Sheet2 Sheet3
10 of 32 records found
NUM
start
Excel Work S...
New Folder
Microsoft Exc...
12:33 PM

Fig. 13

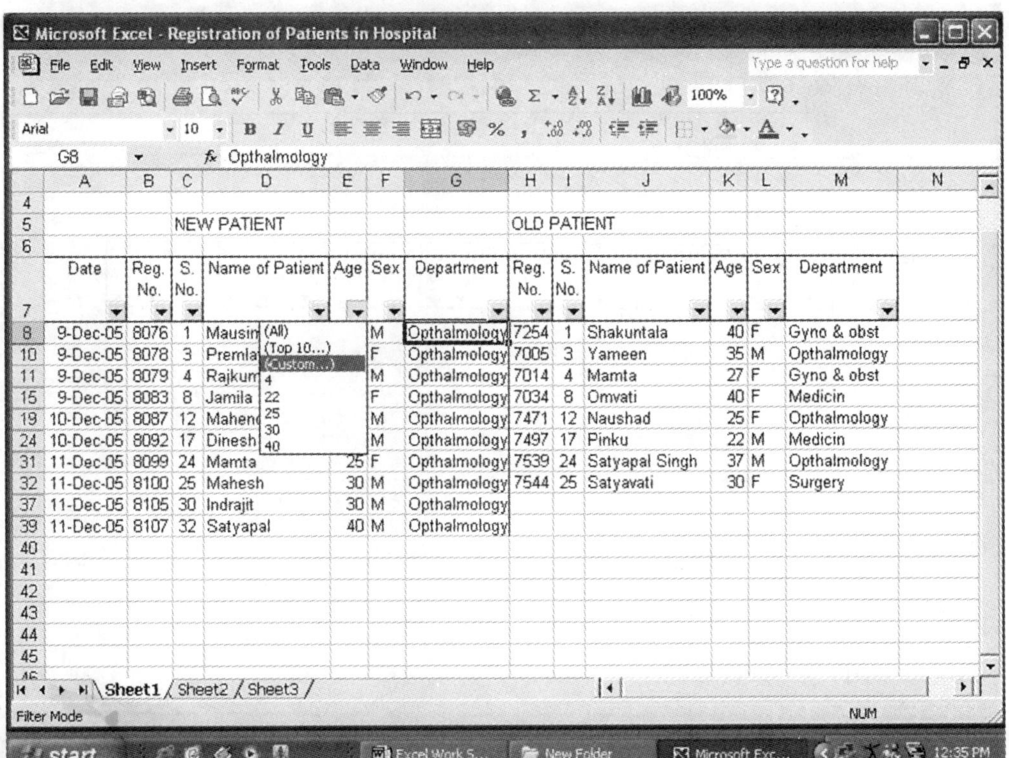
Microsoft Excel - Registration of Patients in Hospital
File Edit View Insert Format Tools Data Window Help
Type a question for help
Arial 10 100%
G8 Opthalmology
NEW PATIENT
OLD PATIENT
Date Reg. No. S. No. Name of Patient Age Sex Department Reg. No. S. No. Name of Patient Age Sex Department
(All)
(Top 10...)
(Custom...)
4
22
25
30
40
Sheet1 Sheet2 Sheet3
Filter Mode
NUM
start
Excel Work S...
New Folder
Microsoft Exc...
12:35 PM

Fig. 14

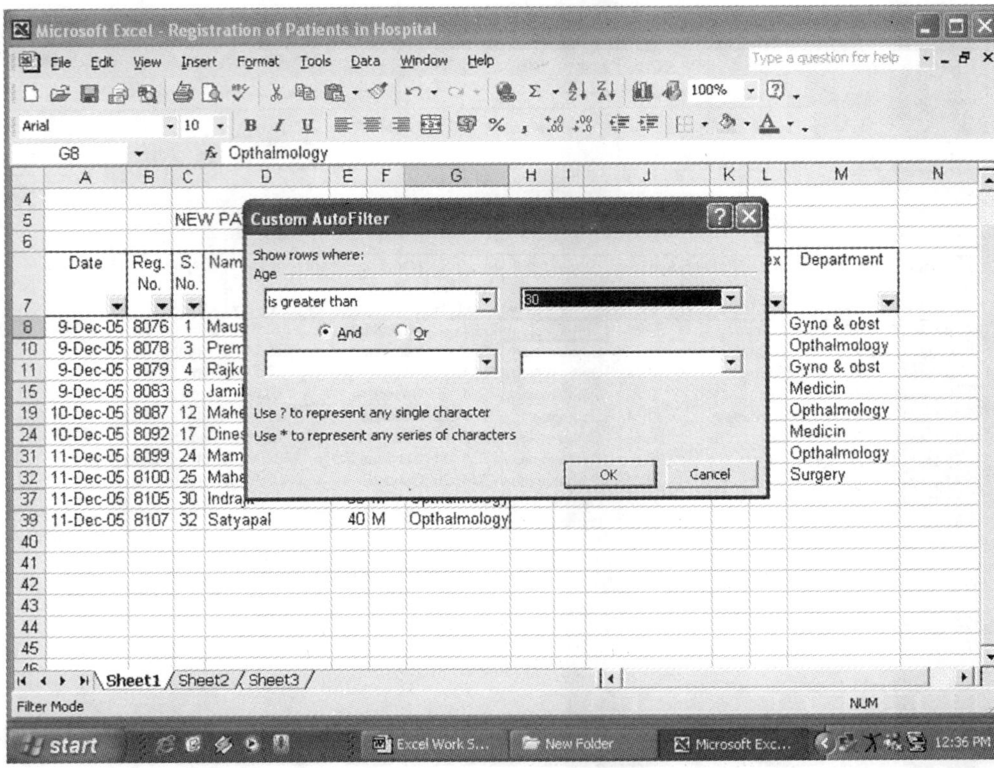
Microsoft Excel - Registration of Patients in Hospital
Custom AutoFilter
Show rows where:
Age
is greater than
30
And
Or
Use ? to represent any single character
Use * to represent any series of characters
OK
Cancel
Filter Mode

Fig. 15

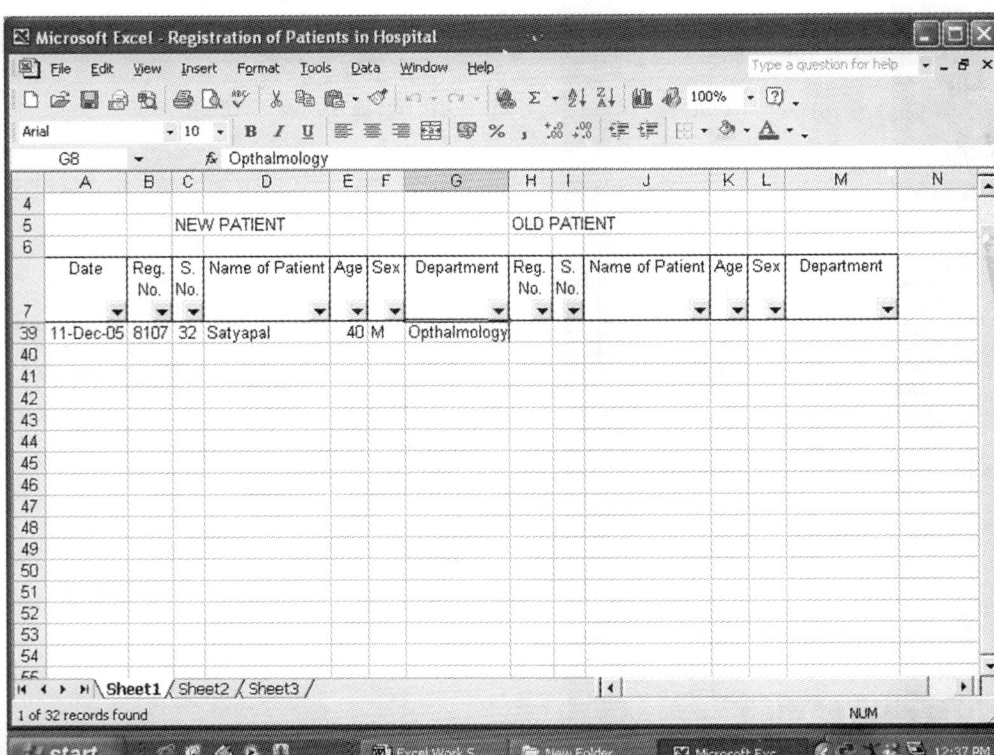
Microsoft Excel - Registration of Patients in Hospital
NEW PATIENT
OLD PATIENT
Date
Reg. No.
S. No.
Name of Patient
Age
Sex
Department
11-Dec-05 8107 32 Satyapal 40 M Opthalmology
1 of 32 records found

Fig. 16